Nonmelanoma Skin Cancer of the Head and Neck

Editor

CEMAL CINGI

FACIAL PLASTIC SURGERY CLINICS OF NORTH AMERICA

www.facialplastic.theclinics.com

Consulting Editor
J. REGAN THOMAS

November 2012 • Volume 20 • Number 4

ELSEVIER

1600 John F. Kennedy Blvd., Suite 1800, Philadelphia, PA 19103-2899

http://www.theclinics.com

FACIAL PLASTIC SURGERY CLINICS OF NORTH AMERICA Volume 20, Number 4
November 2012 ISSN 1064-7406, ISBN 978-1-4557-5871-5

Editor: Joanne Husovski

Facial Plastic Surgery Clinics of North America (ISSN 1064-7406) is published quarterly by Elsevier Inc., 360 Park Avenue South, New York, NY 10010-1710. Months of issue are February, May, August, and November. Business and Editorial Offices: 1600 John F. Kennedy Blvd., Suite 1800, Philadelphia, PA 19103-2899. Periodicals postage paid at New York, NY, and additional mailing offices. Subscription prices are $359.00 per year (US individuals), $496.00 per year (US institutions), $409.00 per year (Canadian individuals), $594.00 per year (Canadian institutions), $489.00 per year (foreign individuals), $594.00 per year (foreign institutions), $170.00 per year (US students), and $237.00 per year (foreign students). Foreign air speed delivery is included in all *Clinics* subscription prices. All prices are subject to change without notice. POSTMASTER: Send address changes to *Facial Plastic Surgery Clinics*, Elsevier Health Sciences Division, Subscription Customer Service, 3251 Riverport Lane, Maryland Heights, MO 63043. **Customer service: 1-800-654-2452 (US and Canada); 1-314-447-8871 (outside US and Canada); Fax: 314-447-8029; E-mail:journalscustomerservice-usa@elsevier.com (for print support); journalsonline support-usa@elsevier.com (for online support).**

Reprints. For copies of 100 or more of articles in this publication, please contact the Commercial Reprints Department, Elsevier Inc., 360 Park Avenue South, New York, NY 10010-1710. Tel.: 212-633-3812; Fax: 212-462-1935; E-mail: reprints@elsevier.com.

Facial Plastic Surgery Clinics of North America is covered in *MEDLINE/PubMed* (*Index Medicus*).

Printed and bound by CPI Group (UK) Ltd, Croydon, CR0 4YY

Transferred to digital print 2012

Contributors

CONSULTING EDITOR

J. REGAN THOMAS, MD, FACS
Professor and Chairman, Department of
Otolaryngology, University of Illinois at
Chicago, Chicago, Illinois

GUEST EDITOR

CEMAL CINGI, MD
Professor, Department of Otorhinolaryngology
Head and Neck Surgery, Eskisehir Osmangazi
University, Eskisehir, Turkey

AUTHORS

PETER ADAMSON, MD
Professor, Adamson Associates Cosmetic
Facial-Head and Neck Surgery Clinic, Toronto,
Canada

TIMUR M. AKCAM, MD
Associate Professor, Department of
Otorhinolaryngology, Gulhane Military Medical
Academy, Ankara, Turkey

SHAN BAKER, MD
Facial Plastic and Reconstructive Surgery,
Department of Otolaryngology Head and Neck
Surgery, University of Michigan, Michigan

BURAK ÖMÜR CAKIR, MD
Associate Professor, Department of
Otorhinolaryngology Head and Neck Surgery,
Sisli Etfal Education and Research Hospital,
Istanbul, Turkey

CEMAL CINGI, MD
Professor, Department of Otorhinolaryngology
Head and Neck Surgery, Eskisehir Osmangazi
University, Eskisehir, Turkey

H. BENGÜ COBANOGLU, MD
Department of Otorhinolaryngology, Kanuni
Education and Research Hospital, Trabzon,
Turkey

MINAS CONSTANTINIDES, MD, FACS
Director of Facial & Reconstructive Surgery,
Assistant Professor, Department of
Otolaryngology, New York University Langone
Medical Center, New York

AYLIN TÜREL ERMERTCAN, MD
Professor, Department of Dermatology,
Faculty of Medicine, Celal Bayar University,
Manisa, Turkey

GÖRKEM ESKIIZMIR, MD
Associate Professor, Department of
Otolaryngology-Head and Neck Surgery,
Faculty of Medicine, Celal Bayar University,
Manisa, Turkey

OREN FRIEDMAN, MD
Director, Facial Plastic Surgery, Associate
Professor, Otolaryngology-Head and Neck
Surgery, University of Pennsylvania,
Philadelphia, Pennsylvania

GULSUM GENCOGLAN, MD
Associate Professor of Dermatology,
Department of Dermatology, Medical Faculty
of Celal Bayar University, Manisa, Turkey

WOLFGANG GUBISCH, MD
Professor, Department of Plastic and
Reconstructive Surgery, Marien Hospital,
Stutgard, Germany

PETER W. HELLINGS, MD
Professor, Department of Otorhinolaryngology,
University Hospitals, Leuven, Belgium

FATIH OGHAN, MD
Assistant Professor, Department of
Otolaryngology, Head and Neck Surgery,
Dumlupinar University, Kutahya, Turkey

FEZAL OZDEMIR, MD
Professor of Dermatology, Department of
Dermatology, Medical Faculty of
Ege University, Izmir, Turkey

DAVID R. REINSTADLER, MD
Department of Otolaryngology–Head and
Neck Surgery, University of Southern
California, Los Angeles, California

UTTAM K. SINHA, MD
Department of Otolaryngology–Head and Neck
Surgery, University of Southern California,
Los Angeles, California

HALIS UNLU, MD
Professor, Department of Otorhinolaryngology,
Head and Neck Surgery, EKOL Hospital, Izmir,
Turkey

AHMET URAL, MD
Associate Professor, Department of
Otolaryngology, Faculty of Medicine,
Karadeniz Technical University, Trabzon,
Turkey

METIN YILMAZ, MD
Professor, Department of Otolaryngology-
Head and Neck Surgery, Gazi University
Hospital, Ankara, Turkey

Contents

but nonsurgical treatment options may be indicated in specific cases. Nonsurgical treatment options for NMSC may be preferred as good alternatives under certain circumstances. This review provides a comprehensive overview of the nonsurgical treatment modalities for NMSCs, such as curettage and electrodesiccation, cryotherapy, radiotherapy, laser, photodynamic therapy, immunotherapy, and retinoid therapy.

This article focuses on the surgical treatment of nonmelanoma skin cancers of the head and neck. The risk factors of nonmelanoma skin cancers for recurrence and metastases that are important for choosing the best treatment option are summarized. Surgical treatment options including surgical excision with standard margins, frozen section, staged surgery, and Mohs micrographic surgery are described. Indications, techniques, outcomes, and advantages and disadvantages of each approach are reviewed. Finally, management of incomplete excisions is discussed.

Although the metastatic rate of cutaneous squamous cell carcinoma (SCC) is low, detailed examination for the presence of micro- and macrometastasis of lymph nodes is crucial in avoiding the devastating outcomes and in planning appropriate treatment. Cutaneous SCC of the head and neck can spread to parotid lymph nodes, cervical lymph nodes, or both, depending on the location of the primary tumor. Therefore, clinical and radiologic evaluation of the parotid and neck should be performed in patients with cutaneous SCC. Optimal treatment of metastatic cutaneous SCC of the head and neck should consist of complete surgical resection with adjuvant radiotherapy.

This article concentrates on the less-common cutaneous malignancies such as merkel cell, atypical fibroxanthoma, malignant fibrous histiocytoma, dermatofibrosarcoma protuberans, microcystic adnexal carcinoma, and sebaceous carcinoma. The clinical and histopathologic descriptions of each, most current and emerging etiologies, diagnosis, staging, treatment, and prognosis are discussed.

Reconstruction of facial defects formed after resection of skin cancers is a challenging procedure. Achieving the best functional and aesthetic outcome depends on accurate preoperative planning. Reconstructive surgeons should perform a detailed analysis of the facial defect based on location, size, and depth and choose the most appropriate technique according to their experiences and patient preferences and expectations. This article reviews the preoperative analysis of facial defects, and the major principles and techniques of facial reconstruction. Discussed are reconstruction of the nose, lip, cheek, forehead, and eyelid, presenting for each technique the goals of the reconstruction, types of flaps and grafts, and surgical technique.

The importance and effectiveness of prevention efforts and strategies for skin cancers are reviewed. Topical sunscreens and their proper use are presented. Topical and ingested forms of natural, synthetic, or biologic chemical agents that are potentially efficacious for chemoprevention are listtdldted and discussed.

Contents

technique, the goals of the reconstruction, types of flaps and grafts, and surgical technique

Fatih Oghan, Gorkem Eskiizmir, Halis Unlu, and Cemal Cingi

The importance and effectiveness of prevention efforts and strategies for skin care are reviewed. Topical sunscreens and their proper use are presented. Topical and possible forms of natural, synthetic, or biologic chemical agents that are potentially efficacious for chemoprevention are listed/tabulated and discussed.

Advisory Board to Facial Plastic Surgery Clinics 2012

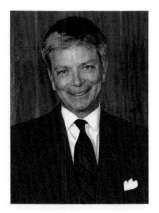
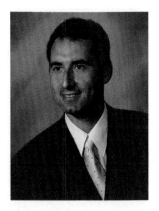
Facial Plastic Surgery Clinics is pleased to introduce the 2012 **Advisory Board**.

Facial Plastic Surgery Clinics is widely available through the media of print, digital e-Reader, online via the Internet, and on iPad and smart phones.

Facial Plastic Surgery Clinics provides professionals access to pertinent point-of-care answers and current clinical information, along with comprehensive background information for deeper understanding.

Readers are welcome to contact the Clinics Editor or Board with comments.

BOARD MEMBERS 2012

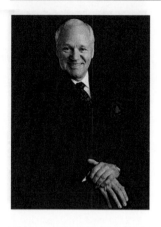

PETER A. ADAMSON, MD

Professor and Head
Division of Facial Plastic and Reconstructive Surgery
Department of Otolaryngology–Head and Neck Surgery
University of Toronto
Toronto, Ontario, Canada

Adamson Cosmetic Facial Surgery
Renaissance Plaza; 150 Bloor Street West; Suite M110
Toronto, Ontario M5S 2X9

416.323.3900
paa@dradamson.com
www.dradamson.com

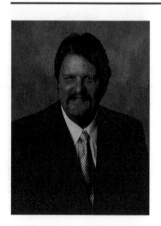

RICK DAVIS, MD

Voluntary Professor
The University of Miami Miller School of Medicine
Miami, Florida

The Center for Facial Restoration
1951 S.W. 172nd Ave; Suite 205
Miramar, Florida 33029

954.442.5191
drd@davisrhinoplasty.com
www.DavisRhinoplasty.com

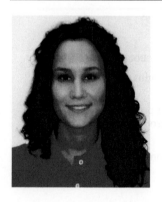

TATIANA DIXON, MD

University of Illinois at Chicago
Resident,
Department of Otolaryngology–Head and Neck Surgery

1855 W. Taylor
Chicago, IL 60612

312.996.6555
TFeuer1@UIC.EDU

STEVEN FAGIEN, MD, FACS

Aesthetic Eyelid Plastic Surgery
660 Glades Road; Suite 210
Boca Raton, Florida 33431

561.393.9898
sfagien@aol.com

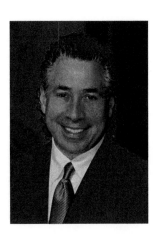

GREG KELLER, MD

Clinical Professor of Surgery, Head and Neck,
David Geffen School of Medicine,
University of California, Los Angeles;

Keller Facial Plastic Surgery
221 W. Pueblo St. Ste A
Santa Barbara, CA 93105

805.687.6408
faclft@aol.com
www.gregorykeller.com

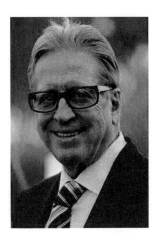

THEDA C. KONTIS, MD

Assistant Professor, Johns Hopkins Hospital
Facial Plastic Surgicenter, Ltd.
1838 Greene Tree Road, Suite 370
Baltimore, MD 21208

410.486.3400
tckontis@aol.com
www.facialplasticsurgerymd.com
www.facial-plasticsurgery.com

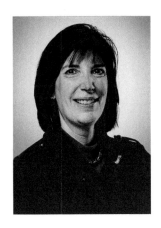

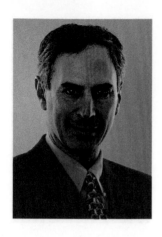

IRA D. PAPEL, MD

Facial Plastic Surgicenter
Associate Professor
The Johns Hopkins University
1838 Greene Tree Road, Suite 370
Baltimore, MD 21208

410.486.3400
idpmd@aol.com
www.facial-plasticsurgery.com

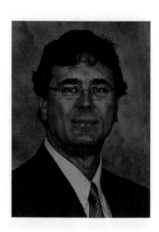

SHERARD A. TATUM, MD

Professor of Otolaryngology and
Pediatrics Cleft and Craniofacial Center
Division of Facial Plastic Surgery
Upstate Medical University
750 E. Adams St.
Syracuse, NY 13210

315.464.4636
TatumS@upstate.edu
www.upstate.edu

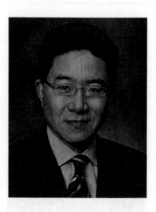

TOM D. WANG, MD

Professor
Facial Plastic and Reconstructive Surgery
Oregon Health & Science University
3181 Southwest Sam Jackson Park Road
Portland, OR 97239

503.494.5678
wangt@ohsu.edu
www.ohsu.edu/drtomwang

FACIAL PLASTIC SURGERY CLINICS OF NORTH AMERICA

Preface
Nonmelanoma Skin Cancer of the Head and Neck

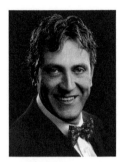

Cemal Cingi, MD
Guest Editor

It has been a great honor for me to be a Guest Editor of this issue, entitled "Nonmelanoma Skin Cancer of the Head and Neck" in *Facial Plastic Surgery Clinics of North America*. Nonmelanoma skin cancers, especially basal cell carcinoma and squamous cell carcinoma, are the most common malignancies with involvement of the head and neck predominantly. Unfortunately, recent investigations and data have emerged indicating the rising incidence and morbidity of nonmelanoma skin cancers worldwide. As a matter of fact, different medical disciplines such as dermatology, otolaryngology, plastic surgery, radiology, and medical oncology all play a role in the diagnosis and medical and surgical treatment of nonmelanoma skin cancers. Therefore, the management of nonmelanoma skin cancers requires a multidisciplinary perspective and close collaboration.

In this issue, the aim is to supply a contemporary reference with completely up-to-date overviews for clinicians and surgeons by reviewing different aspects of nonmelanoma skin cancers of the head and neck. I feel that this issue will be a valuable resource for otolaryngologists, dermatologists, and plastic surgeons. We approach this with a multidisciplinary and international perspective to present several aspects of nonmelanoma skin cancer of the head and neck from different views. In addition, all the topics were rigorously prepared by recognized authors who are experts in their respective surgical, clinical, and research areas. I would like to thank all authors for their insightful contributions to this issue.

Cemal Cingi, MD
Department of Otorhinolaryngology
Head and Neck Surgery
Eskisehir Osmangazi University
Eskisehir, Turkey

E-mail addresses:
ccingi@ogu.edu.tr
ccingi@gmail.com

Facial Plast Surg Clin N Am 20 (2012) xv
http://dx.doi.org/10.1016/j.fsc.2012.08.006
1064-7406/12/$ – see front matter © 2012 Elsevier Inc. All rights reserved.

Nonmelanoma Skin Cancer of the Head and Neck
Current Diagnosis and Treatment

Görkem Eskiizmir, MD[a], Cemal Cingi, MD[b],*

KEYWORDS

- Head and neck cancer • Non melanoma skin cancer • Skin cancer epidemiology
- Skin cancer demographics

KEY POINTS

- Skin cancers, mainly classified as melanoma and nonmelanoma skin cancers (NMSCs), are the most common cancers in humans.
- The most common types of NMSCs are basal cell carcinoma and squamous cell carcinoma.
- Nonmelanoma skin cancers are generally considered as a neglected health problem owing to their low morbidity and mortality; however, the economic burden of health interventions in NMSC is on the increase.
- Patients with a NMSC are generally complained of a nonhealing, ulcerative, and bleeding lesion.
- A dermoscopic examination of a suspicious lesion is helpful for differential diagnosis; and excision or biopsy is generally recommended for histopathological evaluation.
- The gold standard treatment modality for NMSCs is surgical resection.
- Surgical margin control has a paramount importance for decreasing the rate of tumor recurrence.

SKIN CANCER INCIDENCE

Skin cancers are the most common cancers in humans, especially in the white population. They are mainly classified as melanoma and nonmelanoma skin cancers (NMSCs). Unfortunately, the worldwide incidence of NMSCs is not known exactly; they are generally considered a neglected health problem owing to their low morbidity and mortality. Therefore, the cancer registration databases are unreliable even in most of the developed countries; however, evidence demonstrates that the incidence of NMSC has continually and dramatically increased over the past decades in the western world.[1–4] A recent systematic review that evaluated the global incidence for NMSCs determined that Australia has the highest incidence in the world.[5] In 2002, the reported incidence for NMSCs in Australia was 1170/100,000 and the estimated number of patients with NMSCs was 374,000.[3] In addition, the economic burden spent on the care settings and treatment modalities of NMSCs was more than $264 million.[6] Meanwhile, the incidence for NMSCs in the United States cannot be regarded as too low to overlook. In the United States, the estimated total number of new NMSCs was 3,507,693 in 2006, and approximately 3.69 million in 2008.[7,8] The estimated total cost of NMSCs was approximately $426 million per year in the Medicare population.[9] In addition, Guy and Ekwueme[10] reported the years of potential life lost and indirect expenditures of skin cancers (including melanoma and NMSCs), which ranged from $28.9 to $39.2 million for morbidity, and $1.0 to $3.3 billion for mortality. Epidemiologic studies and health economic analysis highlight that the

a Department of Otolaryngology-Head & Neck Surgery, Celal Bayar University, Uncubozköy yerleşkesi, 45030, Manisa, Turkey; b Department of Otorhinolaryngology-Head & Neck Surgery, Eskisehir Osmangazi University, Meşelik Kampüsü, 26480, Eskisehir, Turkey
* Corresponding author.
E-mail address: ccingi@gmail.com

Facial Plast Surg Clin N Am 20 (2012) 415–417
http://dx.doi.org/10.1016/j.fsc.2012.07.003

facialplastic.theclinics.com

incidence of NMSCs is increasing and it is becoming an important public health problem worldwide with an increasing economic impact. Therefore, several countries and the World Health Organization (INTERSUN program) recommend and encourage preventive strategies (eg, sun-protective behaviors and attitudes, topical sunscreens) against skin cancers. In addition, skin cancer screening programs have been implemented recently with promising results in certain countries, such as Germany.[11]

COMMON TYPES OF NONMELANOMA SKIN CANCERS

The most common types of NMSCs are basal cell carcinoma (BCC) and squamous cell carcinoma (SCC), although several other rare types, such as Merkel cell carcinoma and sebaceous gland carcinoma are also present.

The major etiologic factor for the development of NMSCs is overexposure to solar ultraviolet (UV) radiation, especially UVB (ranging 320 to 290 nm). Therefore, the sun-exposed skin regions, such as the head, neck, and extremities, are at higher risk for the development of NMSCs. The development of BCC is associated with *intermittent exposure* to the sun. The development of actinic keratosis (precancerous progenitor of SCC) and/or invasive SCC is associated with *continual, chronic sun exposure*. UV radiation-induced carcinogenesis in NMSCs is basically related to a defect in the repair of UV radiation-induced DNA damage. In BCC, mutations in Hedgehog signaling pathway–related genes, and in SCC, mutations in *p53* tumor suppressor genes play a key role.[12–14]

Basal Cell Carcinoma

Basal cell carcinoma, the most frequent subtype of NMSCs, originates from the basal cells of the epidermis. It almost always invades the local structures; however, it rarely metastasizes. It has various subtypes, which are mainly classified according to their clinical and histopathological characteristics: noduloulcerative, superficial, morpheaform, infiltrative, basosquamous, cystic, and fibroepithelioma of Pinkus. Noduloulcerative and superficial BCC are the most common subtypes and generally involve the head and neck regions. Morpheaform, infiltrative, and basosquamous subtypes of BCC are less commonly detected; however, they have a more aggressive behavior.

Squamous Cell Carcinoma

Squamous cell carcinoma originates from epidermal keratinocytes. It is a locally aggressive skin cancer, which also has the potential to metastasize to regional lymph nodes and distant structures. The incidence of regional lymph node involvement in cutaneous SCC of the head and neck is approximately 5%; and the lymph nodes in the parotid gland are a metastatic basin for cutaneous SCC of the head and neck.[15] Unfortunately, the survival of patients with metastatic cutaneous SCC decreases dramatically (overall 5-year survival rate of 34.4%).[16]

HISTORY AND EXAMINATION FOR NONMELANOMA SKIN CANCERS

Most patients with NMSCs report a history of non-healing, ulcerative, bleeding lesions. In physical examination, typical morphologic appearances of BCC (a firm, "pearly" papule or nodule with telengiectasis) and SCC (a papule, nodule, or plaque with or without hyperkeratosis) can be detected. Moreover, dermoscopic examination of the lesions can be helpful in differential diagnosis.[17] Any lesion with a suspicion of skin cancer should be excised or biopsied for histopathological examination.

TREATMENT FOR NONMELANOMA SKIN CANCERS

The gold standard treatment modality for NMSCs is surgical resection; however, cryotherapy, radiotherapy, curettage and electrodessication, photodynamic therapy, or topical immunmodulators may be recommended as an alternative therapy to patients who are not good candidates for surgery or are unwilling to have a surgical procedure. The major goal of a surgical excision is to have a tumor-free excision area while preserving the maximal healthy tissue. Surgical margin control is of paramount importance in the management of NMSCs. Tumor recurrence is rare (<2%) when a tumor-free surgical margin is achieved; on the other hand, a high rate of tumor recurrence (25%–41%) has been reported in incompletely excised lesions.[18–21]

SURGICAL INTERVENTIONS FOR NONMELANOMA SKIN CANCERS

The surgical interventions for NMSCs are Mohs micrographic surgery, surgical excision with postoperative margin assessment, and surgical excision with complete circumferential peripheral and deep margin assessment with frozen or permanent sections (staged surgery).[18,22] Mohs micrographic surgery is performed successfully for the management of both BCC (1.4% in primary tumors and 4.0% in recurrent tumors) and SCC (2.6% in primary tumors and 5.9% in recurrent tumors) with a very low recurrence rate.[23,24] However, staged surgery with permanent sections may be considered in patients with high-risk NMSCs and recurrent tumor, or after a Mohs micrographic surgery failure.[18,25] A defect is formed after the surgical excision of the tumor. Therefore, a reconstruction technique is generally required to obtain a functional structure and a esthetically pleasant appearance, unless the defect size is small enough for primary closure. A successful facial reconstruction mainly depends on an accurate defect analysis and surgical plan that is tailored according to the size, depth, and location of the defect, and meticulous application of surgery. In addition, a good physician-patient relationship is essential; thereby, patients' expectations can be realized by the surgeon and the details (eg, surgical outcome, complications) about the reconstruction technique can be discussed with the patient preoperatively.

REFERENCES

1. Gloster HM Jr, Brodland DG. The epidemiology of skin cancer. Dermatol Surg 1996;22:217–26.
2. Geller AC, Annas GD. Epidemiology of melanoma and nonmelanoma skin cancer. Semin Oncol Nurs 2003;19:2–11.
3. Staples MP, Elwood M, Burton RC, et al. Non-melanoma skin cancer in Australia: the 2002 national survey and trends since 1985. Med J Aust 2006; 184:6–10.
4. Leiter U, Garbe C. Epidemiology of melanoma and nonmelanoma skin cancer—the role of sunlight. Adv Exp Med Biol 2008;624:89–103.
5. Lomas A, Leonardi-Bee J, Bath-Hextall F. A systematic review of worldwide incidence of nonmelanoma skin cancer. Br J Dermatol 2012;166:1069–80.
6. Australian Institute of Health and Welfare. Health system expenditures on cancer and other neoplasms in Australia, 2000–01. Health and Welfare Expenditure Series No. 22. Canberra (Australia): AIHW; 2005. AIHW Catalogue No. HWE 29.
7. Rogers HW, Weinstock MA, Harris AR, et al. Incidence estimate of nonmelanoma skin cancer in the United States, 2006. Arch Dermatol 2010;146:283–7.
8. Donaldson MR, Coldiron BM. No end in sight: the skin cancer epidemic continues. Semin Cutan Med Surg 2011;30:3–5.
9. Chen JG, Fleischer AB Jr, Smith ED, et al. Cost of nonmelanoma skin cancer treatment in the United States. Dermatol Surg 2001;27:1035–8.
10. Guy GP, Ekwueme DU. Years of potential life lost and indirect costs of melanoma and non-melanoma skin cancer: a systematic review of the literature. Pharmacoeconomics 2011;29:863–74.
11. Breitbart EW, Waldmann A, Nolte S, et al. Systematic skin cancer screening in Northern Germany. J Am Acad Dermatol 2012;66:201–11.
12. Brash DE, Rudolph JA, Simon JA, et al. A role for sunlight in skin cancer: UV-induced p53 mutations in squamous cell carcinoma. Proc Natl Acad Sci U S A 1991;88:10124–8.
13. de Gruijl FR, van Kranen HJ, Mullenders LH. UV-induced DNA damage, repair, mutations and oncogenic pathways in skin cancer. J Photochem Photobiol B 2001;63:19–27.
14. Göppner D, Leverkus M. Basal cell carcinoma: from the molecular understanding of the pathogenesis to targeted therapy of progressive disease. J Skin Cancer 2011;2011:650258.
15. O'Brien CJ. The parotid gland as a metastatic basin for cutaneous cancer. Arch Otolaryngol Head Neck Surg 2005;131:551–5.
16. Rowe DE, Carroll RJ, Day CL. Prognostic factors for local recurrence, metastasis, and survival rates in squamous cell carcinoma of the skin, ear, and lip. J Am Acad Dermatol 1992;26:976–90.
17. Zaballos P, Llambrich A, Puig S, et al. Dermoscopy is useful for the recognition of benign-malignant compound tumours. Br J Dermatol 2005;153: 653–6.
18. Walker P, Hill D. Surgical treatment of basal cell carcinomas using standard postoperative histological assessment. Australas J Dermatol 2006;47:1–12.
19. Sherry KR, Reid LA, Wilmshurst AD. A five year review of basal cell carcinoma excisions. J Plast Reconstr Aesthet Surg 2010;63:1485–9.
20. Sussman LA, Liggins DF. Incompletely excised basal cell carcinoma: a management dilemma? Aust N Z J Surg 1996;66:276–8.
21. De Silva SP, Dellon AL. Recurrence rates of positive margin basal cell carcinoma: results of a five year prospective study. J Surg Oncol 1985;28:72–4.
22. Cumberland L, Dana A, Liegeois N. Mohs micrographic surgery for the management of nonmelanoma skin cancers. Facial Plast Surg Clin North Am 2009;17:325–35.
23. Leibovitch I, Huilgol SC, Selva D, et al. Cutaneous squamous cell carcinoma treated with Mohs micrographic surgery in Australia. I. Experience over 10 years. J Am Acad Dermatol 2005;53:253–60.
24. Leibovitch I, Huilgol SC, Selva D, et al. Basal cell carcinoma treated with Mohs surgery in Australia. II. Outcome at 5-year follow-up. J Am Acad Dermatol 2005;53:452–7.
25. Eskiizmir G, Gençoglan G, Temiz P, et al. Staged-surgery with permanent pathology for the management of nonmelanoma skin cancer of the nose. Eur Arch Otorhinolaryngol 2011;268:117–21.

Epidemiology and Economic Burden of Nonmelanoma Skin Cancer

Burak Ömür Cakir, MD[a], Peter Adamson, MD[b],
Cemal Cingi, MD[c],*

KEYWORDS

- Head and neck cancer • Non melanoma skin cancer • Skin cancer costs
- Skin cancer epidemiology • Healthcare costs

KEY POINTS

- The prevalence of skin cancer cases is approximately 5 times higher than the prevalence of breast or prostate cancer and higher than the prevalence of all other cancers.
- Australia has the highest incidence of skin cancer in the world, and nonmelanoma skin cancer (NMSC) is the most commonly diagnosed cancer in Australia.
- NMSC in the United States is primarily treated by dermatologists, but also by general surgeons, plastic surgeons, facial plastic surgeons, otolaryngologists, and radiation oncologists.
- Major environmental and risk factors for NMSC are frequent exposure to ultraviolet radiation or sunlight, thinning of the ozone layer, immune suppression, increased life longevity, mutations in the PTCH gene, and fair skin.

Skin cancer includes 2 large groups: cutaneous melanoma and nonmelanoma skin cancer (NMSC).

Nonmelanoma skin cancer is the most common form of cancer in the world and approximately 40% of all malignancies. The incidence of nonmelanoma skin cancer has increased since the 1990s, but its mortality rate has decreased. The following are major environmental and risk factors for NMSC:

- Frequent exposure to ultraviolet (UV) radiation or sunlight
- Thinning of the ozone layer
- Immune suppression
- Increased life longevity
- Mutations in the PTCH gene
- Fair skin

UV radiation is considered to be the most important factor for the development of skin cancer. NMSC is seen mostly in men and generally appears in older patients, but the incidence in young women

has increased because of lifestyle changes, related to clothing and increased sun exposure. NMSC is usually located on sun-exposed areas of the body. These carcinomas are seen mostly on the head, neck, trunk, and the limbs.[1,2]

The term NMSC refers to 2 different conditions: basal cell carcinoma (BCC) and squamous cell carcinoma (SCC).

1. BCC grows slowly and is rarely fatal. If it is not detected early, it can damage the surrounding tissue and bones.
2. SCC is more invasive and it is more likely to damage the surrounding tissue and to metastasize. If it is caught early, SCC is highly treatable.

INCIDENCE OF NONMELANOMA SKIN CANCER

The registration of incidence rates of NMSC is likely not correct because NMSC is considered

a Department of Otorhinolaryngology and Head Neck Surgery, Sisli Etfal Education and Research Hospital, Istanbul, Turkey; b Adamson Associates Cosmetic Facial-Head and Neck Surgery Clinic, Toronto, Canada; c Department of Otorhinolaryngology and Head Neck Surgery, Eskisehir Osmangazi University, Eskisehir, Turkey
* Corresponding author.
E-mail address: ccingi@gmail.com

Facial Plast Surg Clin N Am 20 (2012) 419–422
http://dx.doi.org/10.1016/j.fsc.2012.07.004
1064-7406/12/$ – see front matter © 2012 Elsevier Inc. All rights reserved.

a negligible health problem with low risks of mortality and morbidity. NMSC is curable when it is detected early and appropriately treated; it can also be prevented through protective measures. Therefore, it is important to determine the number of cases in the population. We do know that NMSC is the most common cancer affecting Caucasians, with the incidence increasing worldwide. Australia has the highest incidence of skin cancer in the world; the population-based cancer registry shows that, in Australia, the incidence of this cancer type has increased 1.5-fold over the past 17 years.[2] The incidence of BCC is higher than SCC and the rates in men are higher than women for both cancer types. In 2002, the age-standardized rate per 100,000 population for NMSC was 1170, the rates of BCC were 884, and for SCC were 387.[3] The approximate number of NMSC patients in Australia was 374,000 and an estimated 2% of the Australian population is treated for these cancers each year. The rates increase with age. Four percent of the affected population is older than 40 years and 8% are older than 70. Multiple primary NMSCs are seen frequently. Approximately 40% of cases can develop a second NMSC within 2 years.[4]

NMSC is also the most common malignancy in the United States; however, the exact incidence of NMSC is unknown because NMSC is not reported in most registries. A mathematical model was used to estimate the prevalence of NMSC in the United States. The number of procedures for NMSC among Medicare patients increased 76.9% between 1992 and 2006, from 1,158,298 to 2,048,517. From 2002 to 2006 the number of NMSCs increased 16%; the estimated total number of NMSCs in the United States in 2006 was 3,507,693 and the total number of people treated for NMSC was 2,152,500.[5] Using mathematical research from the National Health Interview Survey, 2007, and the National Cancer Institute Skin Cancer Incidence Data (1977–1978), it is estimated that 13 million white non-Hispanic individuals in the United States in 2007 had a history of at least 1 NMSC and 1 in 5 people aged 70 years or older was diagnosed with NMSC.[6]

No reliable epidemiologic data exist for NMSC in most European Union countries because these low-grade carcinomas are not recorded. Studies show that in Europe, there was an increase of the incidence of NMSC during the 25-year period between 1978 and 2002. Women were more affected with NMSC, and the highest rate was obtained in Switzerland (Geneva) between 1998 and 2002. The incidence rate was found to be 113 per 100,000. In men, the highest incidence was observed in Ireland, with an incidence rate of 146 per 100,000 persons. In Europe, the highest incidence was observed in Switzerland and Ireland.[7] The average incidence rates in England were 76 of 100,000 persons for BBC and 22 of 100,000 persons for SCC.[8]

HEALTH CARE COSTS OF NONMELANOMA SKIN CANCER

The increasing incidence of NMSC has an important impact on health care costs. Skin cancer has the potential to lead to years of potential life lost and lost productivity. Findings from a study estimated the average number of years of potential life lost per death for NMSC of 10.[9] The prevalence of skin cancer cases is approximately 5 times higher than the prevalence of breast or prostate cancer and higher than the prevalence of all other cancers.[6] Compared with other cancer types, NMSC treatment costs are currently low because NMSC can be primarily treated efficiently in office-based settings. NMSC care cost stands in fifth place after prostate, lung, colon, and breast carcinomas. Cost of NMSC care depends on 2 factors: care settings and treatment modalities.[10,11] Treatment modalities include surgical excision, microscopically controlled surgical excision (Mohs surgery), radiation therapy electrodessication, curettage, cryosurgery, laser ablation photodynamic therapy, and topical chemotherapeutic agents.[12]

NMSC IN THE UNITED STATES

In the United States, the total cost of NMSC care in the Medicare population is $426 million per year. Care settings for NMSC include hospitals, outpatient departments, ambulatory surgical centers, and physician offices. NMSC is mostly treated by dermatologists but also by general surgeons, plastic surgeons, facial plastic surgeons, otolaryngologists, and radiation oncologists.[13] The cost per episode of care in a physician's office setting is approximately $492, which in this setting it provided the lowest cost per episode of care.[10] The comparative costs per episode of care in inpatient and outpatient settings were $5537 and $1043, respectively.[14] Regarding the treatment modalities of NMSC, Mohs micrographic surgery was shown to be similar in cost to traditional surgical excision and less costly than excision with frozen sections. Electrodessication and curettage was reported as a less costly procedure. The problem for surgical excision is the necessity for a second procedure in 32% to 39% of cases to obtain clear margins.[10] The percentages of care procedures were found range between 9.6% and

41.0% for Mohs surgery, 40.0% to 75.8% for excision, and 14.4% to 19.0% for electrodessication and curettage.[13,15] A positive correlation was found between cost and tumor size. The cost per episode also varies depending on tumor location.[10,14] The cost is higher if the tumor is located on the feet, neck, face, ear, or eyelids. The mean cost ranges from $384 to $1097.[14] The cost for NMSC was reported as $28.9 million for morbidity and $1 billion for mortality in the United States.[9]

NMSC IN AUSTRALIA

As mentioned, Australia has the highest incidence of skin cancer in the world, and NMSC is the most commonly diagnosed cancer in Australia. In Australia, from 2000 to 2001, the estimated cost of NMSC was $264 million, which was 9% of the total costs for all types of cancer treatment.[16] New Zealand and Australia have the same incidence of NMSC, the estimated number of cases being treated in New Zealand annually being 80,000. The estimated cost is more than NZ $50 million per year.[2] The Australian government's Strengthening Cancer Care initiative has reserved more than $189.4 million over 5 years to decrease the burden of cancer. The purpose of this political decision was to provide better coordination of the national cancer effort through increased research for cancer care, cancer prevention and screening program, and better support and treatment procedures. It was the most comprehensive skin cancer prevention program created in the world.[17]

NMSC IN EUROPE

NMSC is also an economic burden to the health system in Europe. In the United Kingdom, the estimated number of NMSC cases annually is 78,370. The cost per case for NMSC is £889. In 2006, the total cost of skin cancer in England was estimated to be more than £270 million; 45% of the total cost of skin cancer was attributable to NMSC. The estimated costs for the National Health Service were £112.4 million (42%). The remaining costs were attributed to the patient's own costs, morbidity and mortality costs.[18] In Germany in 2003, in patients aged 90 years or older, 14% of all cancer-related hospitalizations were attributable to NMSC, and the number of cases was 41,929. The estimated annual hospitalization cost in Germany was €105 to €130 million.[19] In Sweden, the corresponding cost for inpatient care of NMSC was approximately €3928 per patient. The total cost for inpatient care attributable to NMSC represented approximately €5.2 million. The corresponding cost for outpatient care of NMSC was approximately €549 per patient. Health care costs and lost productivity were €36.2 million.[20]

WORLDWIDE NMSC

The number of NMSC cases increased dramatically between 1990 and 2010. Because of this, NMSC presents an increasing problem for health care services worldwide. The costs attributable to related health care procedures and lost productivity is now an economic burden and will likely become an increased one. Unfortunately, the exact incidence is unknown because of incomplete registration of cases in most countries. It is important that the incidence of NMSC be better determined so that prevention strategies can be planned and the most cost-effective treatment modalities established. Health care providers everywhere should be promoting the establishment of appropriate registries to ultimately improve the preventive provision of care for NMSC.

REFERENCES

1. Nyugen TH, Ho DD. Nonmelanoma skin cancer. Curr Treat Options Oncol 2002;3:193–203.
2. Brougham ND, Dennett ER, Tan ST. Non-melanoma skin cancers in New Zealand—a neglected problem. N Z Med J 2010;123:59–65.
3. Staples MP, Elwood M, Burton RC, et al. Non-melanoma skin cancer in Australia: the 2002 national survey and trends since 1985. Med J Aust 2006;184:6–10.
4. Raasch BA, Buettner PG. Multiple nonmelanoma skin cancer in an exposed Australian population. Int J Dermatol 2002;41:652–8.
5. Rogers HW, Weinstock MA, Harris AR, et al. Incidence estimate of nonmelanoma skin cancer in the United States, 2006. Arch Dermatol 2010;146:283–7.
6. Stern RS. Prevalence of a history of skin cancer in 2007: results of an incidence-based model. Arch Dermatol 2010;146:283–7.
7. Madera PA, Eisman AB, Santiago SA, et al. Changes in the incidence of skin cancer between 1978-2002. Actas Dermosifiliogr 2010;101:39–46.
8. Lomas A, Leonardi-Bee J, Bath-Extall F. A systematic review of worldwide incidence on non-melanoma skin cancer. Br J Dermatol 2012;166(5):1069–80.
9. Guy GP, Ekwueme DU. Years of potential life lost and indirect costs of melanoma and non-melanoma skin cancer: a systematic review of the literature. Pharmacoeconomics 2011;29:863–74.
10. Mudigonda T, Pearce DJ, Yentzer BA, et al. The economic impact of non-melanoma skin cancer: a review. J Natl Compr Canc Netw 2010;8:888–96.
11. Housman TS, Feldman SR, Williford PM, et al. Skin cancer is among the most costly of all cancers to

treat for the Medicare population. J Am Acad Dermatol 2003;48:425–9.

12. Tierney EP, Hanke CW. Cost effectiveness of Mohs micrographic surgery: review of the literature. J Drugs Dermatol 2009;8:914–22.

13. Chen GJ, Yelverton CB, Polisetty SS, et al. Treatment patterns and cost of nonmelanoma skin cancer management. Dermatol Surg 2006;32: 1266–71.

14. Chen GJ, Fleischer AB, Smith ED, et al. Cost of nonmelanoma skin cancer treatment in the United States. Dermatol Surg 2001;27:1035–8.

15. Asgari MM, Bertenthal D, Sen S, et al. Patient satisfaction after treatment of nonmelanoma skin cancer. Dermatol Surg 2009;35:1041–9.

16. Health system expenditures on cancer and other neoplasms in Australia, 2000-01. Canberra (Australia): Australian Institute of Health and Welfare; 2005. Report No.: 22.

17. Australian Government Department of Health and Ageing. Health Fact Sheet 1-Investing in Australia's health: strengthening cancer care, Available at: http://www.health.gov.au/internet/budget/Publishing. nsf/Content/health-budget2005-hbudget-hfact1.htm. Accessed November 22, 2005.

18. 2004-2006 Data from National Clinical and Health Outcomes Knowledge Base of UK, (NCHOD).

19. Stang A, Stausberg J, Boedeker W, et al. Nationwide hospitalization costs of skin melanoma and nonmelanoma skin cancer in Germany. J Eur Acad Dermatol Venereol 2008;22:65–72.

20. Tinghög G, Carlsson P, Synnerstad I, et al. Societal Cost of Skin Cancer in Sweden in 2005. Acta Derm Venereol 2008;88:467–73.

Nonmelanoma Skin Cancer of the Head and Neck
Clinical Evaluation and Histopathology

Gulsum Gencoglan, MD[a],*, Fezal Ozdemir, MD[b]

KEYWORDS

- Skin cancer • Actinic keratosis • Bowen's disease • Basal cell carcinoma
- Squamous cell carcinoma • Pathology • Dermoscopy • Reflectance confocal microscopy

KEY POINTS

- In most nonmelanoma skin cancer (NMSC) tumors, diagnosis is easy for their typical morphologic appearance; however, it is sometimes difficult to differentiate the pigmented or nonpigmented skin lesions clinically.
- With the naked eye, only half of pigmented lesions are correctly diagnosed; dermoscopy increases the diagnostic sensitivity to 95%.
- Besides diagnosis, dermoscopy and confocal microscopy have the advantage of selection of location for biopsy, determination of appropriate therapeutic modalities, verification of treatment efficacy, and decision of surgical margins.
- The central zone of the face, temples, lips, ears, and the scalp have significant risk for local recurrence and metastases of squamous cell carcinoma (SCC). Similar to basal cell carcinoma, the growth of SCC tends to follow the regions of the least resistant, spreading along the perichondrium, periosteum, fascia, and embryonic fusion planes.

INTRODUCTION

Nonmelanoma skin cancer (NMSC) is the most common skin cancer affecting both sexes. In most of these tumors, diagnosis is easy for their typical morphologic appearance[1]; however, it may sometimes be difficult to differentiate the pigmented or nonpigmented skin lesions clinically.

Dermoscopy is a practical technique for the evaluation of pigmented and nonpigmented skin lesions, including melanoma and NMSC. It is a noninvasive and inexpensive in vivo tool that permits the visualization of morphologic features that are not visible to the naked eye.[2] With the naked eye, only half of the pigmented lesions are correctly diagnosed.[3] Dermoscopy, which is useful in the differential diagnosis of melanocytic and nonmelanocytic lesions, increases the diagnostic sensitivity to 95%.[4,5] A 10-fold magnification is generally sufficient for the assessment of the suspicious skin lesions, but magnifications up to ×100 are possible.[6]

Reflectance confocal microscopy (RCM) is a new optical method that is useful for obtaining the detailed images of tissue architecture and cellular morphology of living tissues. It does not need fixation, sectioning, and staining, but provides in near real-time imaging with a high resolution and contrast.[7] In contrast to vertical sections in histologic evaluation, RCM obtains horizontal (en face) optical sections in gray scale.[8] These horizontal images of the skin at the cellular

a Department of Dermatology, Celal Bayar University, 45050, Manisa, Turkey; b Department of Dermatology, Ege University, 35100, Izmir, Turkey
* Corresponding author.
E-mail address: gencoglan75@hotmail.com

Facial Plast Surg Clin N Am 20 (2012) 423–435
http://dx.doi.org/10.1016/j.fsc.2012.07.005
1064-7406/12/$ – see front matter © 2012 Elsevier Inc. All rights reserved.

resolution can be viewed from the surface down to 150 μm, which is the depth of the papillary dermis.[9] A digital camera connected to the RCM computer obtains dermoscopic images directly correlated with RCM evaluation and guides the identification of suspicious areas within the lesion.[8] RCM has been used for the evaluation of a variety of inflammatory and neoplastic skin disorders.[9,10]

Although these 2 easy methods are useful for clinicians in the diagnosis and follow-up, histopathological evaluation is still the gold standard; however, the 2 methods decrease unnecessary excision rates and are useful in the monitoring of the new lesions and recurrences. Here, clinical, histopathologic, dermoscopic, and RCM features of NMSC are reviewed.

BASAL CELL CARCINOMA
Clinical Findings in Basal Cell Carcinoma

Basal cell carcinoma (BCC) has clinical variants that are nodulo-ulcerative, morpheaform, infiltrative, superficial, basosquamous, cystic, and fibroepitheliomatous. The most common type, nodular BCC, occurs mainly on the face as a firm, "pearly" papule or nodule with a telengiectasic surface. In time, the dome-shaped lesions tend to be eroded and ulcerated.[1] Nodular BCC accounts for 75% to 80% of all cases (**Fig. 1**).[11] Approximately 90% of nodular BCCs are found on the head and neck. These may be heavily pigmented because of the presence of melanin, so that it is sometimes impossible to exclude melanoma by only visual inspection (**Fig. 2**). The superficial type of BCC is the second common subtype of BCC (15%), which mainly affects the trunk and the extremities; however, it can be localized on the head and neck area also (**Fig. 3**).[12]

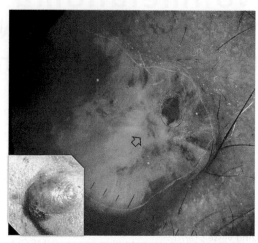

Fig. 2. Pigmented nodular BCC; ulceration (*circle*), arborizing vessels (*arrow*), irregular scattered gray dots and globules (*asterisk*).

The less common infiltrative (**Fig. 4**) and morpheaform (**Fig. 5**) types can be seen as poorly defined, lightly pigmented, indurated, flat skin lesions, occasionally with overlying telangiectasia.[13] The lesion may also appear scarlike without a history of skin injury. The head and neck are involved in 95% of these cases. The overlying skin surface may be atrophic, ulcerated, or relatively normal in appearance.

Basosquamous BCC, described as metatypical BCC, is a rare subtype, and is intermediate to nodulocystic BCC and squamous cell carcinoma (SCC) (**Fig. 6**).[12]

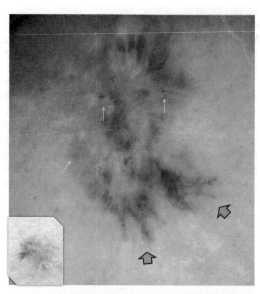

Fig. 3. Superficial BCC; brown/gray leaf-like areas (*blue arrows*) and globules (*white arrows*).

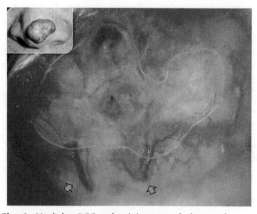

Fig. 1. Nodular BCC; arborizing vessels (*arrows*).

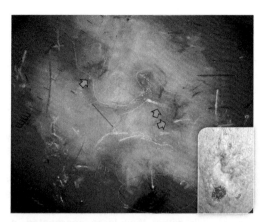

Fig. 4. Infiltrative BCC; ulceration (*circle*) and arborizing vessels (*arrows*).

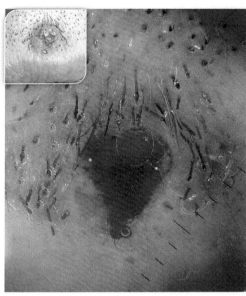

Fig. 6. Basosquamous BCC; blue/gray blotch (*asterisks*), polymorphous vessels (*circle*).

Cystic types have a clear or blue-gray appearance and exude a clear fluid if punctured or cut. If the lesion is in the periorbital area, it may be confused with a hidrocystoma. Cystic degeneration in a BCC is not often obvious clinically, thus the lesion may sometimes appear as a typical nodular BCC (**Fig. 7**).

Fibroepithelioma of Pinkus is a rare variant of BCC, which usually presents as a smooth pinkish nodule or plaque on the lower back. It may be difficult to distinguish it clinically from amelanotic melanoma, but it has unique histologic features. Sometimes it may be pedunculated.[14]

BCCs are typically slow-growing lesions up to 1 or 2 cm in diameter. BCC usually remains local and almost never spreads to other parts of the body; however, it may invade nearby tissues and structures, including the nerves, bones, and brain, especially the histologically aggressive subtypes. Metastases of BCC are rare, occurring in only 0.003% to 0.05% of patients, and most commonly occur via the lymphatics to the regional nodes.[11]

Histologic subtype of the tumor, age of the patient, and the anatomic location are the most important factors in identifying high-risk BCC. The midface region, which comprises the nasal dorsum, nasal tip, nasal ala, nasolabial folds, philtrum, inner canthus, and forehead, seems to have the highest recurrence rate. The auricular and periauricular areas are the next most frequent sites for recurrence. All these preferred anatomic sites are because of an increased UV exposure. The skin and subcutaneous tissue in these areas are relatively thin, which permits tumor spreading along the periosteum and perichondrium. The

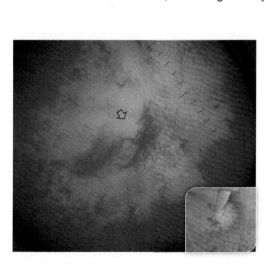

Fig. 5. Morpheaform BCC; arborizing vessels (*arrow*).

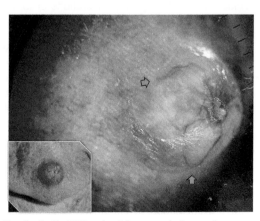

Fig. 7. Cystic BCC; arborizing vessels (*arrows*).

embryologic fusion planes in these regions also provide easy paths for spreading.[13]

Histopathology of BCC

BCC is an adnexal tumor composed of tumor nests with aggregates of basaloid cells and characteristic palisading. The peripheral cells surround the less-organized cells in the center of tumor nests. The nuclei of tumor cells are generally uniform and hyperchromatic, and the cytoplasm is scanty and poorly demarcated.[14]

BCC has distinct histologic types, like its clinical variants. Any histologic variant may be locally aggressive and metastasize, but those with basosquamous, morpheaform, infiltrating, and micronodular growth patterns seem to do so more frequently. Some of the most important subtypes listed as follows are selected either because of their frequency of occurrence or their aggressive nature.

The cell clusters are composed of rounded and bluntly branched lobules of small hyperchromatic cells, which are connected to the overlying epidermis by narrow cords or broad trabeculae. The tumor cells are uniform in size and polygonal in shape, with generally oval nuclei and inconspicuous nucleoli. The nuclei of the peripheral cells of the clusters are aligned in parallel and at right angles to those in the center of the nodules; so-called "peripheral palisading." Another common finding is retraction artifact, or "cleft formation," which is the result of shrinkage of mucin during tissue fixation and staining. Zero to 2 mitotic figures are typically seen per high-power field, but up to 10 may be observed in selected cases. Peritumoral actinic elastosis is almost invariably seen in the surrounding dermis. Not uncommonly, centrilobular necrosis in nodular BCCs accounts for their cystic quality. The overlying epidermis may or may not be ulcerated.[15]

The histologic characteristics of superficial BCC include buds and irregular proliferations of tumor cells attached to atrophic epidermis, and they show little or no penetration into the dermis.[16]

The morpheaform type is named so because of the densely collagenized, hypocellular fibrous matrix that is an integral part of its growth pattern. Inflammation is characteristically sparse or absent, and palisading is not present. The connection between the tumor and epidermis is usually focal. Morpheaform BCC is characterized by its deep invasion of the dermis. The overlying skin surface may be atrophic, ulcerated, or relatively normal.[17]

Infiltrative BCC lesions are hybrids of the nodular and morpheaform types in that they show a combination of expansive solid cellular, branched, sharply angulated, and linear cell groups. These lesions lack a central cohesive mass and have a distinctive fibroblast-rich stroma. Although virtually all BCCs permeate the dermis and, hence, are "infiltrative" by definition, the term infiltrative BCC is reserved for this aggressive histologic subtype that can expand both peripherally (like morpheaform subtypes) and show deep extension to underlying soft tissue.[18]

The micronodular type is considered biologically distinct from other subtypes of BCC because of its high propensity for local recurrence. Similar to infiltrating BCC, these lesions have the propensity for dispersion of the nests of epithelial cells. These neoplasms are made of small, round aggregates of basal cells rather than large aggregates, as seen in solid BCCs.[18,19]

Basosquamous BCC includes distinct but admixed components of BCC and overt SCC. The distinction between these lesions and SCC is that they retain the typical organization of basal cell carcinoma, that is, islands of epithelial cells embedded in a fibrovascular stroma.[20]

Dermoscopic Findings in BCC

In most cases, the diagnosis is easy with the typical morphologic appearance; however, it is sometimes difficult to differentiate pigment-containing BCCs from melanomas because of their asymmetric pigmentation. Dermoscopy is a practical tool for the evaluation of pigmented skin lesions in routine clinical examination. This technique is important especially in the diagnosis of an early melanoma. Various dermoscopic criteria have been identified in the differential diagnosis of melanocytic or nonmelanocytic pigmented skin lesions.[21] Menzies[22] described the criteria for the dermoscopic diagnosis of pigmented BCCs: the absence of a pigment network and the presence of at least 1 of 6 positive morphologic features: ulceration, multiple blue-gray globules (see **Figs. 2** and **3**), leaflike areas (see **Fig. 3**), arborizing vessels (see **Figs. 1, 2, 4, 5** and **7**), large blue-gray ovoid nests, and spoke wheel areas.

The presence of arborizing vessels is the dermoscopic hallmark of pigmented BCC and can be appreciated even better in the nonpigmented nodular type (see **Fig. 1**). Dermoscopic examination of these lesions is recommended, especially when the differentiation from SCC and keratoacanthoma is difficult on clinical grounds. The latter ones are characterized by hairpin vessels surrounded by a whitish halo (dermoscopic sign of keratinization) and dotted vessels (**Figs. 8** and **9**), whereas BCC nearly exclusively displays arborizing vessels (**Table 1**).[2] Pigmented BCC also

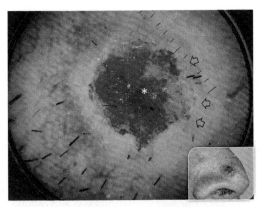

Fig. 8. SCC; hairpin vessels surrounded by a whitish halo (*arrows*) and polymorphous vessels (*asterisk*).

sometimes can be difficult to distinguish clinically from melanoma. Besides the pathognomonic vascular pattern consisting of vessels with different diameters and numerous branches, leaf-like areas with an opaque gray-brown to slate-gray pigmentation, mostly situated at the periphery of the lesion, represent additional dermoscopic clues for the diagnosis of BCC.[22] However, only gray dots/globules and irregularly outlined gray structures are sometimes visible. In conjunction with the complete absence of other melanoma-specific dermoscopic criteria, these gray structures may lead to the diagnosis of BCC.[21] Menzies' method gives an overall sensitivity of 93% for BCC and specificity of 89% using

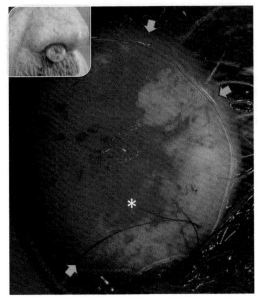

Fig. 9. Keratoacanthoma; hairpin vessels (*arrows*) and polymorphous vessels (*asterisk*).

the invasive melanoma set.[22] Dermoscopy showing the characteristic criteria for pigmented BCC plays an important role in diagnosis.

Reflectance Confocal Microscopy for BCC

BCC is generally considered to be the most common primary malignant neoplasm in human beings. Because they grow exceedingly slowly, most BCCs are innocuous; however, if they are not treated properly, they can cause extensive local tissue destruction, and may lead to death by infiltrating and destroying vital structures.[15] Therefore, clinical monitoring of tumor persistence or recurrence after the treatment is important. Where local recurrence or persistence is suspected, biopsy is generally required for the diagnostic confirmation. Dermoscopic examination in monitoring treatment response may be limited if scarring is present. At this point, RCM may be useful.

RCM can detect specific BCC features that correlate with histopathology. The clinical application of this technique showed excellent diagnostic accuracy for the diagnosis of BCC. In the epidermis, a streaming pattern of elongated monomorphic keratinocyte nuclei that are polarized along one axis on the background of variable epidermal disarray is a feature often found. In the papillary dermis, cell aggregations with a nodular/cordlike growth pattern can be seen, as well as peritumoural dark cleftlike spaces.[23] These are consistent with the basaloid aggregations of a BCC that often display the typical palisading of tumor cell nuclei, and the latter represents peritumoural mucinous edema. The vascular pattern has been reported to play an important diagnostic role. Vessels that are branched and orientated parallel to the horizontal surface have been described in BCCs. Inflammatory infiltrate and the presence of bright dendritic cells and melanophages (in pigmented BCC) are also often observed.[9] With its relatively high correlation with standard microscopy findings, RCM has been used to assess treatment responses to imiquimod and photodynamic therapy.[24,25] Similarly, RCM imaging of shave biopsy wounds is feasible and demonstrates the future possibility of intraoperative mapping in surgical wounds.[26]

ACTINIC KERATOSIS

Actinic keratosis (AK) has been characterized as benign "precancerous" or "premalignant" because the atypical keratinocytes within these lesions are confined to the epidermis. There is no risk of metastasis until these lesions evolve into invasive carcinoma.[14]

Table 1
Diagnostic findings of NMSC

	Clinic	Pathology	Dermoscopy	RCM
Basal cell carcinoma	Pearly papule/nodule with pigmentation, ulceration, or scarlike features	Basaloid cell islands in the dermis and palisatic arrangement of tumor cells, peritumoral cleft formation	Arborizing vessels, multiple blue-gray globules, leaflike and spoke-wheel areas and ulceration	Basaloid aggregations, typical palisading of tumor cells and peritumoural dark cleftlike spaces
Actinic keratosis	Multiple discrete, flat or elevated, keratotic plaques	Aggregates of atypical, pleomorphic keratinocytes at the basal layer that may extend upward to involve the granular and cornified layers	Red pseudonetwork pattern and white keratotic hair follicle openings, white/yellow surface scales, linear or wavy vessels	Atypical keratinocytes, nuclear and cellular pleomorphism, hyperkeratosis, parakeratosis, blood vessel dilation and solar elastosis
Bowen disease	Slowly enlarging, flat, pink, scaly patch or plaque	Proliferation of atypical, pleomorphic keratinocytes involving the whole epidermis	Glomerular vessels and a scaly surface, sometimes irregular pigment globules	Atypical honeycomb pattern with great variations in cell and nuclear morphology and whole thickness of the epidermis
Squamous cell carcinoma	Sharply demarcated pink plaques often with ulceration and multiple actinic keratoses	Crowded keratinocytes, atypical mitosis, loss of maturation, nuclear pleomorphism, dyskeratotic cells extension in the dermis	Typically polymorphous blood vessels on center of the lesion, surrounded by whitish halo with hairpin vessels and scales	Atypical cobblestone or honeycomb patterns at the epidermis with a proliferation of atypical keratinocytes

Data from Zalaudek I, Argenziano G, Di Stefani A, et al. Dermoscopy in general dermatology. Dermatology 2006;212:7–18.

Clinical Findings in AK

Any region of the body can be affected if enough actinic damage occurs. Thus, the most common locations are the face and the back of the hands. Lesions are rarely solitary. The presence of other signs of sun-damaged skin, such as solar elastosis or irregular pigmentation, should suggest a fertile field for AK. Visual inspection is best performed with simultaneous palpation to detect lesions. They are usually asymptomatic, although occasional lesions may itch when inflamed.[1] Tenderness on palpation should alert the clinician to the possibility that the lesion has evolved into carcinoma.[14]

As the AKs become somewhat more prominent, they may assume a variety of clinic patterns, described as follows.

Erythematous or atrophic
Early lesions frequently have a pink or red hue and have telangiectases, presumably reflecting the limited inflammatory response.

Keratotic
This is the most common variant. As lesions grow, the normal process of cornification is disrupted and scales accumulate. The color switches from pink to dirty yellow or brown (**Fig. 10**). The extreme variant of the keratotic type is cutaneous horn.

Lichen planus–like
Some lesions, especially those of the dorsal aspect of forearms and chest, may have a purple hue and resemble lichen planus. Histologically they show a lichenoid infiltrate.

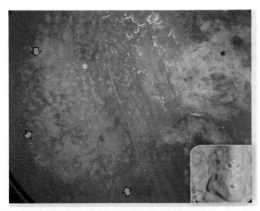

Fig. 10. Keratotic-type actinic keratosis; light brown pseudonetwork and strawberry pattern (*white asterisk*), white/yellow surface scales (*black asterisk*), linear vessels surrounding the hair follicles (*arrows*).

Pigmented

The most common site for the pigmented variant is the face, especially the temples and the cheeks. It is usually light brown, reflecting both a thickened stratum corneum and increased melanin. Changes in melanocytes are not seen. It can be difficult to separate pigmented AK from flat seborrheic keratosis or solar lentigo. If pigmentation is irregular, lentigo maligna must be excluded.

Cheilitis

AK of the lip is almost always localized on the lower lip. The risk of malignant degeneration is somewhat greater than cutaneous lesions.[1]

Histopathology of AK

Several histologic variants have been described, including pigmented, acantholytic, atrophic, bowenoid, lichenoid, hypertrophic, and actinic cheilitis types. All are characterized by atypical keratinocytic proliferation confined to the epidermis.

Histopathologic changes consist of partial-thickness keratinocytic atypia displaying nuclear pleomorphism and disordered maturation from small basal keratinocytes to progressively flattening squame at upper epidermal levels. The lesion may be acanthotic often with increased numbers of buds protruding into the papillary dermis, or atrophic, with loss of rete ridges. The basal layer often appears more basophilic than normal, a consequence of crowding of atypical keratinocytes. Hyperkeratosis and parakeratosis are seen. Acrosyringia and acrotrichia are usually uninvolved. This pattern, characterized by alternating orthokeratosis and parakeratosis, is referred to as the "flag sign." AK is almost always associated with solar elastosis in the dermis.[14]

The answer to the histologic question of when AK starts to become an SCC is a partly subjective decision made by the dermatopathologist. Diagnosis of early or microinvasive SCC arising in AK is probably the best solution when only occasional malignant cells are present in the papillary dermis, as it warns the clinician that this particular lesion requires special attention. When islands or strands of malignant keratinocytes are present in the dermis, then the diagnosis should be SCC.[1]

Dermoscopic Findings in AK

Dermoscopically, facial AKs commonly reveal a red pseudonetwork pattern and white keratotic hair follicle openings, the "strawberry pattern," white/yellow surface scales, linear or wavy vessels surrounding the hair follicles, and yellowish keratotic plugs (see **Fig. 10**). The strawberry pattern consists of an erythema forming a marked pink-to-red "pseudonetwork" around the hair follicles. This pattern is found in more than 90% of lesions.[27]

Some special AK subtypes may reveal different patterns. For example, Bowenoid AK is typified by glomerular (linear coiled) vessels, which are regularly distributed and not arranged in clusters, as seen in classic Bowen disease (BD) (**Fig. 11**). Hyperkeratotic AK frequently shows surface scale and erythema (see **Fig. 10**).[28]

Pigmented AK is often characterized by lack of associated erythema and has a hyperpigmented or reticulated appearance. If pigmentation is irregular, it can be difficult to discriminate pigmented AK from flat seborrheic keratosis, solar lentigines, and early melanomas. Dermoscopy may be

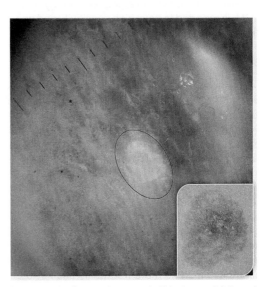

Fig. 11. BD; glomerular vessels (*black asterisks*), scale (*circle*).

a useful adjunct in these situations. On the face, they may exhibit a particular pigmented pseudo-network.[29] This pseudonetwork refers to a network of pigment that may be formed when closely set follicular openings spared of pigment are found within a background of a pigmented epidermis; this dermoscopic finding has been referred to as a "pseudonetwork" because the network itself is not a manifestation of hyperpigmented rete ridges, as in a conventional pigment network. In addition, various subpatterns have been delineated that are frequently encountered for these pigmented lesions found on the face. The presence of asymmetric pigmented follicules, annular granular pigment pattern, or rhomboid pigment pattern, or a combination of these, should lower the threshold to biopsy to exclude a melanoma. Dermoscopic examination enables the recognition of these subtle pigment patterns attributable to these common pigmented lesions, providing additional morphologic features in assessing the pigmented lesions of the face.[30]

Reflectance Confocal Microscopy for AK

Besides the characteristic features of actinic keratosis, subclinical AK can be detected by RCM also, leading to the early identification of affected sites and better therapeutic efficacy.[31] The most frequently defined RCM features of AK include stratum corneum disruption, epidermal pleomorphism, and architectural disarray of the epidermis.[32,33] The diagnosis of AK is generally based on clinical examination; however, biopsy and histologic evaluation are performed in clinically indistinct cases and if invasive SCC is suspected. However, noninvasive imaging technology, in vivo RCM, is reported to have high sensitivity and specificity rates for diagnosis and follow-up.[31]

BOWEN DISEASE
Clinical Findings in Bowen Disease

Bowen disease (BD) is a malignant intraepithelial tumor that affects older adults, especially women. Typically, it presents as a slowly enlarging, flat, pink, scaly patch or plaque on lower extremities, face, and intertriginous areas (see **Fig. 11**). It may rarely be pruritic. Occasionally annular lesions or more bizarre patterns evolve and the central parts may appear to involute. Contiguous lesions can intersect and form polycyclic designs. The presence of an ulceration or nodule suggests the development of an invasive tumor.[1] The pigmented variant of BD is rare. Pigmented BD has been described as more frequently seen in dark-skinned individuals.[34] It should be differentiated from other pigmented lesions, such as seborrheic

keratosis, pigmented AK, solar lentigo, pigmented and superficial BCC, melanocytic nevus, blue nevus, melanoma, keratoacanthoma, angioma, and angiokeratoma.[28,35,36] Differential diagnosis is easy by dermoscopy. Biopsy and pathologic examination should be performed for suspicious lesions.[36]

Histopathology of BD

BD is a form of epidermal carcinoma in situ, characterized histologically by proliferation of atypical, pleomorphic keratinocytes involving the whole epidermis. In addition, the epidermal pattern is altered. There is acanthosis, and the rete ridges are larger and more bulbous. Dyskeratotic, mitotic and multinucleated cells frequently occur. There may be a brisk inflammatory response in the epidermis consisting of lymphocytes and plasma cells.[1]

Dermoscopic Findings in BD

Dermoscopy has been used for the diagnosis of pigmented and nonpigmented BD, showing a peculiar pattern characterized by glomerular vessels and a scaly surface in 100% and 90% of cases, respectively (see **Fig. 11**).[34] In addition to these dermoscopic clues, pigmented BD may exhibit irregular pigment globules in a patchy distribution, gray-brown homogeneous pigmentation, and pseudonetwork. Glomerular vessels are larger than dotted vessels, regular and arranged in clusters. The linear arrangement of glomerular vessels is a specific clue to BD.[37] Regular dotted vessels can also be found in psoriasis, viral warts, and clear cell acanthoma; however, psoriasis and warts are easy to differentiate by clinical examination, and clear cell acanthoma has a linear or string of "pearls" pattern to the dotted vessels. Amelanotic melanoma can also have dotted vessels, but linear arrangement of vessels and presence of keratin can help to distinguish them. In contrast to other pigmented lesions, the dermoscopy of pigmented BD is not specific, and the diagnosis is often a difficult one. It is a keratinous tumor, and therefore scaly surface has been reported as a dermoscopic hallmark in 90% of cases of BD, and most pigmented BD. It can be a diagnostic clue to distinguish from other pigmented skin lesions, such as pigmented BCC and melanoma.[28,36] Scaly surface corresponds to a hyperkeratotic and parakeratotic stratum corneum.[37]

Reflectance Confocal Microscopy for BD

There is only one report in the literature about the reflectance confocal microscopic features of BD. The investigators report that an atypical honeycomb pattern with great variations in cell and nuclear morphology is seen at the granular/spinous layers of the epidermis. Within this pattern, 2 types of targetoid cells are observed: the first type, large cells with a bright center and a dark peripheral halo, and the second type, cells with a dark center and a bright rim surrounded by a dark halo. In the center of the dermal papillae, round-to-oval blood vessels with increased tortuosity were observed in all cases. Blood vessels showed a round-to-oval shape within the superficial papillary dermis, but became S-shaped at the level of the lower papillary dermis.[38]

The differential diagnosis of BD includes other nonmelanoma skin cancers and inflammatory dermatoses such as eczema or psoriasis; 0.3% to 5.0% of cases of BD may progress into invasive SCC.[38] Even though the differential diagnosis of BD can be readily made by dermoscopy, the diagnosis is usually based on the histologic examination.

SQUAMOUS CELL CARCINOMA
Clinical Findings in SCC

SCC presents with various clinical appearances. Clinical lesions of SCC in situ range from ill-defined, rough, pink patches similar to AK, to sharply demarcated verrucous papules or plaques. The typical SCC is a skin-colored papule, nodule, or plaque localized on the sun-damaged skin. It may be hyperkeratotic with central necrosis or bleeding (see **Fig. 8**). The biologic behavior differs by the location, size, depth, and grade of histologic differentiation.[1]

The central zone of the face, temples, lips (**Fig. 12**; see **Fig. 8**), ears, and the scalp have significant risk for local recurrence and metastases.[39] Similar to BCC, the growth of SCC tends to follow the regions of least resistance. It prefers to spread along the perichondrium, periosteum, fascia, and embryonic fusion planes.

Perineural invasion (PNI) is seen in 5% to 14% of SCCs of the head and neck,[40,41] whereas in BCC, the rate is 1% to 6%.[42] It is most common in the auricular area (25.7%), cheek and maxilla (21.4%), and the forehead (18.6%).[40] The nerves adjacent to the lesions are most likely to be involved. Cranial nerve involvement can be evaluated by computerized tomography and/or magnetic resonance imaging to demonstrate the enlargement of skull base foramina, and enhancement of major nerve trunks or nerve enlargement.[43] There may be regions of PNI interrupted by normal tissue, namely "skip lesions" for several centimeters. Thus, in the presence of PNI, most investigators recommend aggressive surgical resection, including craniofacial resection if applicable and/or postoperative radiation.[43]

Verrucous carcinoma is a massive, well-differentiated variant of SCC in which the proliferating tumor is large, pale, and glassy with an infiltrating invasive edge; however, this term is incorrectly used for any SCC that has a warty appearance. Cytologic atypia is minimal in this variant. It can be associated with human papilloma virus, and a distinction between a verrucous carcinoma and large wart may be difficult. The difference mainly depends on the massiveness and depth of the lesion. Verrucous carcinoma is usually locally destructive, but does not metastasize.[14] Two-thirds of cases involve the buccal mucosa, and most of the others affect the gingiva. Early lesions are white patches or plaques; however, as they grow, they thicken with protuberant papules and irregular indurated borders (**Fig. 13**). Sometimes the multiple initial lesions may

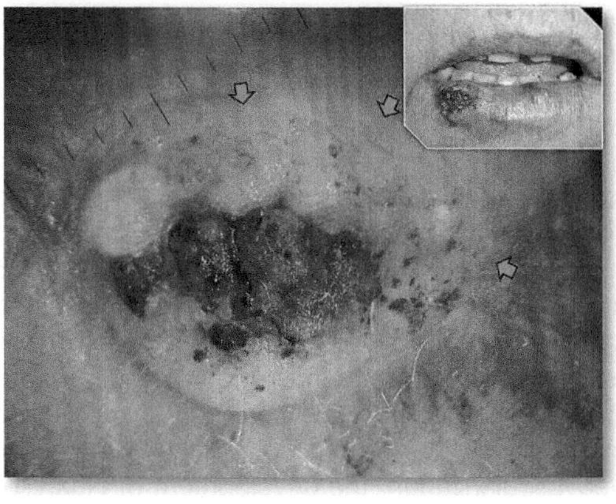

Fig. 12. SCC on the lip; hairpin vessels surrounded by a whitish halo (*arrows*).

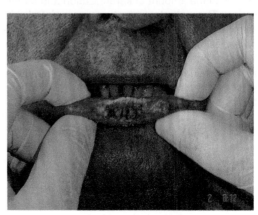

Fig. 13. Verrucous carcinoma on the lip: verrucous, hyperkeratotic, papillomatous projections arising on a white patch.

coalesce. They may grow slowly, but may become large enough to interfere with eating or speaking.[1]

Keratoacanthoma is characterized by its volcano architecture. The tumor is composed of well-differentiated keratinocytes with a brightly eosinophilic glassy cytoplasm surrounding a core filled with cornified material (see **Fig. 9**). An inflammatory infiltrate of lymphocytes and eosinophils is usually present. Small intratumoral abscesses of neutrophils are common. Elastic fibers are often seen within the epithelium at the base.

As the lesion regresses, the dome-shaped architecture flattens and fibrosis develops at the base. Cytologic atypia is minimal. If hyperchromatic nuclei or abnormal mitoses are prominent, it is diagnosed as an ordinary invasive SCC.[14]

Histopathology of SCC

The histologic spectrum of SCC begins with AK. Histologically, the difference among AK, SCC in situ, and frank SCC is described as follows: AK involves only part of the epidermis, SCC in situ occupies the full thickness of the epidermis, and invasive SCC penetrates the basement membrane of the epidermis.[44] As the cells progress from basal to superficial layer, regular maturation is lost, showing variability in nuclear size, shape, and staining; mitotic figures; multinucleation; and usually together with hyperkeratosis and/or parakeratosis. AK is defined as a precursor of SCC, and studies have shown that most cases of SCC arise from AK.[45]

The typical histologic characteristics of SCC include interanastomosing growth of cords and nests of polygonal cells, with eosinophilic or amphophilic cytoplasm, enlarged nuclei, and prominent nucleoli. There is usually a large amount of atypical mitotic figures. This differentiation correlates with the amount of keratinization and cornification. The pathologic features associated with aggressive behavior include the size, depth, site of the lesion, and differentiation. When the tumor size is greater than 2 cm or has a poor differentiation, the recurrence rate is doubled and the metastatic rate is tripled.[39] Tumors with a depth greater than 4 mm have higher metastatic rate.

Differentiation of the SCC is also an important concept. Well-differentiated SCC has an abundant keratin, glassy eosinophilic cytoplasm, and intercellular bridges on high-power microscopy. In addition, there is an irregular infiltration of the dermis by neoplastic keratinocytes at the base of the tumor, and variable degrees of mixed inflammation and fibrosis beneath the lesion. Moderately differentiated SCC is more deeply invasive and manifests more nuclear hyperchromasia and mitotic activity.

Invasion of blood vessels and perineural sheaths may be appreciated. Poorly differentiated squamous carcinoma commonly infiltrates the subcutis and has scant keratinization. Lymphatic and perineural invasion may be observed in approximately 50% of cases.

Spindle and pleomorphic SCC variants are composed exclusively of fusiform and giant pleomorphic cells, with little or no keratinization,[46] such that they resemble sarcomas on conventional morphologic evaluation. Similar to other poorly differentiated cutaneous squamous neoplasms, deep infiltration of the dermis, subcutis, and underlying fascia is frequently observed.[13]

Dermoscopic Findings of SCC

AK usually presents as multiple scaly, reddish macules or papules on sun-exposed sites and are traditionally diagnosed by clinical appearance alone (see **Fig. 10**). Although intraepidermal carcinoma, also called in situ SCC, typically presents as a slowly growing, scaly plaque and invasive SCC as a fast-growing, tender, indurated papule or nodule, differentiation of early lesions from AK on clinical grounds alone can be difficult. Furthermore, other lesions, such as seborrheic keratosis and metaplastic BCC, may at times clinically mimic AK, intraepidermal carcinoma, and invasive SCC. This may cause a delay in the accurate diagnosis of intraepidermal carcinoma or invasive SCC and/or problems in the choice of appropriate treatment, especially in patients with many AK.[47] Only a few studies to date have focused on the dermatoscopic patterns associated with keratinocytic skin cancers, such as nonpigmented AK,[48] intraepidermal carcinoma,[29,48] and invasive SCC.[48]

There are significant differences in the dermoscopic patterns of AK, intraepidermal carcinoma, and invasive SCC and these differences may assist in their clinical diagnosis and subsequent management.

Progression of AK into intraepidermal carcinoma and invasive SCC can be observed on dermatoscopic examination. Initially, AK shows a red pseudonetwork: the "strawberry pattern." The first step of progressing toward intraepidermal carcinoma is characterized by progressive development of a red starburst pattern and yellow-white opaque scales. Initially, the scales are discrete; however, with further progression to intraepidermal carcinoma, they become thicker and coalesce to be located in a predominantly central position. Also, increased neovascularization, the development of clustered dotted/glomerular vessels, can be seen (see **Figs. 8 and 12**). Further steps toward invasive SCC are characterized by progressive development of elongated vessels, keratinization, and ulceration.[47]

Dermatoscopy may aid in the differentiation of facial AK from in situ and potentially invasive SCC, leading clinicians to diagnose in situ or invasive lesions at an early stage, and also to improve the selection of lesions requiring biopsy or excision for definitive histopathologic diagnosis.

Reflectance Confocal Microscopy in SCC

Atypical cobblestone or honeycomb patterns are identified at the epidermis with the proliferation of atypical keratinocytes in SCC. Similarly, the nuclear enhancement of atypical keratinocytes allows the assessment of cellular criteria similar to those used in histopathology, such as nuclear crowding and pleomorphism of size.

In RCM examination, scale crust is present at the level of the stratum corneum and granular spinous layer. At the spinous-granular layer, there is an atypical honeycomb pattern with heterogeneity in the brightness and width of the grid and in the size of the nuclei, suggesting keratinocytic atypia with pleomorphism. Single, round cells with a bright rim and central dark nucleus are seen and these cells are thought to be most consistent with dyskeratotic keratinocytes.[38,49]

Both AKs and SCCs display a loss of the normal honeycomb pattern on RCM as a result of pleomorphism and atypia of keratinocytes: AKs show milder atypia and only in part of the lesion as assessed on RCM mosaic, whereas SCCs show more pronounced atypia or complete loss of the honeycomb pattern (disarranged pattern) and does so in the entire area of the lesion.[26] Reliable differentiation of AK and in situ SCCs from invasive SCCs remains challenging.[7,26,31] Intraoperative margin mapping can further accelerate the procedure without waiting for frozen pathology before proceeding with further surgery.[26]

Diagnosis Summary of Nonmelanoma Skin Cancers

In most of these tumors, diagnosis is easy for the typical morphologic appearance; however, it is sometimes difficult to differentiate the pigmented or nonpigmented skin lesions clinically. Dermoscopy is a practical technique for the evaluation of these lesions and has advantages of being an in vivo, noninvasive, and inexpensive technique with an increased diagnostic sensitivity up to 95% compared with the naked eye. It also decreases the number of excisions of benign lesions, and provides the early diagnosis of NMSC. Confocal scanning laser microscopy was introduced as a novel technique that enables the in vivo examination of the skin at a nearly histologic resolution in various skin disorders, including NMSC. Besides

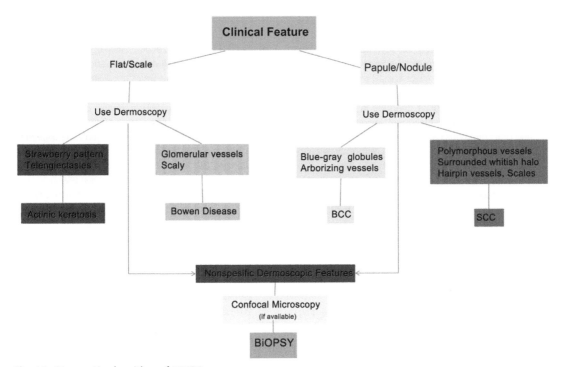

Fig. 14. Diagnostic algorithm of NMSC.

the diagnosis, both of these modalities have other various potential advantages, including selection of location for biopsy, determination of appropriate therapeutic modalities, verification of treatment efficacy, and decision of surgical margins. For the diagnosis of nonmelanoma skin cancer, physical examination is the most critical step, then comes the dermoscopic evaluation. Histopathological examination is mandatory if the lesion is still doubtful. See **Fig. 14** for a diagnostic algorithm for skin cancer.

REFERENCES

1. Sterry W, Stockfleth E. Malignant epithelial tumors. In: Burgdorf WH, Plewig G, Wolff HH, et al, editors. Braun-Falco's dermatology, vol. 96, 3rd edition. Berlin: Springer; 2009. p. 1357–73.

2. Zalaudek I, Argenziano G, Di Stefani A, et al. Dermoscopy in general dermatology. Dermatology 2006; 212:7–18.

3. Kittler H, Pehamberger H, Wolff K, et al. Diagnostic accuracy of dermoscopy. Lancet Oncol 2002;3: 159–65.

4. Argenziano G, Fabbrocini G, Carli P, et al. Epiluminescence microscopy for the diagnosis of doubtful melanocytic skin lesions: comparison of the ABCD rule of dermatoscopy and a new 7-point checklist based on pattern analysis. Arch Dermatol 1998; 134(12):1563–70.

5. Argenziano G, Soyer HP, Chimenti S, et al. Dermoscopy of pigmented skin lesions: results of a consensus meeting via the Internet. J Am Acad Dermatol 2003; 48(5):679–93.

6. Senel E. Dermatoscopy of non-melanocytic skin tumors. Indian J Dermatol Venereol Leprol 2011; 77(1):16–21.

7. Anuthama K, Sherlin HJ, Anuja N, et al. Characterization of different tissue changes in normal, betel chewers, potentially malignant lesions, conditions and oral squamous cell carcinoma using reflectance confocal microscopy: correlation with routine histopathology. Oral Oncol 2010;46(4):232–48.

8. Scope A, Ardigo M, Marghoob AA. Correlation of dermoscopic globule-like structures of dermatofibroma using reflectance confocal microscopy. Dermatology 2008;216:81–2.

9. Wurm EM, Curchin CE, Lambie D, et al. Confocal features of equivocal facial lesions on severely sun-damaged skin: four case studies with dermatoscopic, confocal, and histopathologic correlation. J Am Acad Dermatol 2012;66(3):463–73.

10. Langley RG, Walsh N, Sutherland AE, et al. The diagnostic accuracy of in vivo confocal scanning laser microscopy compared to dermoscopy of benign and malignant melanocytic lesions: a prospective study. Dermatology 2007;215:365–72.

11. Von Domarus H, Steven PJ. Metastatic basal cell carcinoma: report of five cases and review of 170 cases in the literature. J Am Acad Dermatol 1984; 10:1043–60.

12. Scrivener Y, Grosshans E, Cribier B. Variations of basal cell carcinomas according to gender, age, location and histopathological subtype. Br J Dermatol 2002;147(1):41–7.

13. McGuire JF, Ge NN, Dyson S. Nonmelanoma skin cancer of the head and neck I: histopathology and clinical behavior. Am J Otolaryngol 2009;30(2): 121–33.

14. Rigel DS, Cockerell CJ, Carucci J, et al. Actinic keratosis, basal cell carcinoma and squamous cell carcinoma. In: Bolognia JL, Jorizzo JL, Rapini RP, editors. Dermatology, vol. 107, 2nd edition. Spain: Elsevier; 2008. p. 1627–61.

15. Reifenberger J, Ruzicka T. Basal cell carcinoma. In: Burgdorf WH, Plewig G, Wolff HH, et al, editors. Braun-Falco's dermatology, vol. 95, 3rd edition. Berlin: Springer; 2009. p. 1348–56.

16. Bastiaens MT, Hoefnagel JJ, Bruijn JA, et al. Differences in age, site distribution, and sex between nodular and superficial basal cell carcinoma indicate different types of tumors. J Invest Dermatol 1998;110(6):880–4.

17. Teo WL, Wong CH, Song C. Morpheaform facial basal cell carcinoma—a 16-year experience in an Asian center. Int J Dermatol 2011. http://dx.doi.org/10.1111/j.1365–4632.2010.04767.

18. Betti R, Radaelli G, Bombonato C, et al. Anatomic location of basal cell carcinomas may favor certain histologic subtypes. J Cutan Med Surg 2010;14(6): 298–302.

19. Lang PG Jr, Maize JC. Histological evolution of recurrent basal cell carcinoma and treatment implications. J Am Acad Dermatol 1986;14:186–96.

20. DeFaria JL. Basal cell carcinoma of the skin with areas of squamous cell carcinoma: a basosquamous cell carcinoma? J Clin Pathol 1985;38:1273–7.

21. Johr R, Soyer HP, Argenziano G, et al. The essentials of dermoscopy. London: Mosby; 2004. p. 107–39.

22. Menzies SW. Dermoscopy of pigmented basal cell carcinoma. Clin Dermatol 2002;20(3):268–9.

23. Nori S, Rius-Diaz F, Cuevas J, et al. Sensitivity and specificity of reflectance-mode confocal microscopy for in vivo diagnosis of basal cell carcinoma: a multicentre study. J Am Acad Dermatol 2004;51:923–30.

24. Webber SA, Wurm EM, Douglas NC, et al. Effectiveness and limitations of reflectance confocal microscopy in detecting persistence of basal cell carcinomas: a preliminary study. Australas J Dermatol 2011;52(3):179–85.

25. Astner S, Swindells K, Gonzalez S, et al. Confocal microscopy: innovative diagnostic tools for monitoring of non-invasive therapy in cutaneous malignancies. Drug Discov Today 2008;5:81–91.

26. Scope A, Mahmood U, Gareau DS, et al. In vivo reflectance confocal microscopy of shave biopsy wounds: feasibility of intraoperative mapping of cancer margins. Br J Dermatol 2010;163(6):1218–28.

27. Peris K, Micantonio T, Piccolo D, et al. Dermoscopic features of actinic keratosis. J Dtsch Dermatol Ges 2007;5:970–6.

28. Zalaudek I, Leinweber B, Citarella L, et al. Dermoscopy of Bowen's disease. Br J Dermatol 2004; 150:1112–6.

29. Bowling J, Argenziano G, Azenha A, et al. Dermoscopy key points: recommendations from the international dermoscopy society. Dermatology 2007; 214:3–5.

30. Zalaudek I, Kreusch J, Giacomel J, et al. How to diagnose nonpigmented skin tumors: a review of vascular structures seen with dermoscopy: part II. Nonmelanocytic skin tumors. J Am Acad Dermatol 2010;63(3):377–86.

31. Ulrich M, Krueger-Corcoran D, Roewert-Huber J, et al. Reflectance confocal microscopy for noninvasive monitoring of therapy and detection of subclinical actinic keratoses. Dermatology 2010;220(1):15–24.

32. Ulrich M, Maltusch A, Rius-Riaz F, et al. Clinical applicability of in vivo reflectance confocal microscopy for the diagnosis of actinic keratoses. Dermatol Surg 2008;34(5):610–9.

33. Aghassi D, Anderson RR, Gonzalez S. Confocal laser microscopic imaging of actinic keratoses in vivo: a preliminary report. J Am Acad Dermatol 2000;43:42–8.

34. Stante M, De Giorgi V, Massi D, et al. Pigmented Bowen's disease mimicking cutaneous melanoma: clinical and dermoscopic aspects. Dermatol Surg 2004;30(4):541–4.

35. Zalaudek I, Citarella L, Soyer HP, et al. Dermoscopy features of pigmented squamous cell carcinoma: a case report. Dermatol Surg 2004;30(4):539–40.

36. Gutiérrez-Mendoza D, Narro-Llorente R, Karam-Orantes M, et al. Dermoscopy clues in pigmented Bowen's disease. Dermatol Res Pract 2010;2010. pii: 464821.

37. Cameron A, Rosendahl C, Tschandl P, et al. Dermatoscopy of pigmented Bowen's disease. J Am Acad Dermatol 2010;62(4):597–604.

38. Ulrich M, Kanitakis J, González S, et al. Evaluation of Bowen disease by in vivo reflectance confocal microscopy. Br J Dermatol 2012;166(2):451–3.

39. Rowe DE, Carroll RH, Day CL. Prognostic factor for local recurrence, metastasis, and survival rates in squamous cell carcinoma of the skin, ear, and lip. J Am Acad Dermatol 1992;26:976–90.

40. Leibovitch I, Huilgol SC, Selva D, et al. Cutaneous squamous cell carcinoma treated with Mohs micrographic surgery in Australia. II. Perineural invasion. J Am Acad Dermatol 2005;53(2):261–6.

41. Williams LS, Mancuso AA, Mendenhall WM. Perineural spread of cutaneous squamous and basal cell carcinoma: CT and MR detection and its impact on patient management and prognosis. Int J Radiat Oncol Biol Phys 2001;49(4):1061–9.

42. Ratner D, Lowe L, Johnson TM, et al. Perineural spread of basal cell carcinomas treated with Mohs micrographic surgery. Cancer 2000;88(7):1605–13.

43. Backous DD, DeMonte F, El-Naggar A, et al. Craniofacial resection for nonmelanoma skin cancer of the head and neck. Laryngoscope 2005;115(6):931–7.

44. Cassarino DS, Derienzo DP, Barr RJ. Cutaneous squamous cell carcinoma: a comprehensive clinicopathologic classification—part two. J Cutan Pathol 2006;33(4):261–79.

45. Czarnecki D, Meehan CJ, Bruce F, et al. The majority of cutaneous squamous cell carcinomas arise in actinic keratoses. J Cutan Med Surg 2002;6(3):207–9.

46. Marsden JR, Newton-Bishop JA, Burrows L, et al. Revised UK guidelines for the management of cutaneous melanoma 2010. Br J Dermatol 2010;163:238–56.

47. Zalaudek I, Giacomel J, Schmid K, et al. Dermatoscopy of facial actinic keratosis, intraepidermal carcinoma, and invasive squamous cell carcinoma: a progression model. J Am Acad Dermatol 2012; 66(4):589–97.

48. Felder S, Rabinovitz H, Oliviero M, et al. Dermoscopic differentiation of a superficial basal cell carcinoma and squamous cell carcinoma in situ. Dermatol Surg 2006;32:423–5.

49. Braga JC, Scope A, Klaz I, et al. The significance of reflectance confocal microscopy in the assessment of solitary pink skin lesions. J Am Acad Dermatol 2009;61(2):230–41.

Nonmelanoma Skin Cancer of the Head and Neck
Molecular Mechanisms

H. Bengü Cobanoglu, MD[a],*, Minas Constantinides, MD[b],
Ahmet Ural, MD[c]

KEYWORDS

- Molecular • Genetic • Cancer genetics • Carcinogenesis • Ultraviolet radiation
- Hedgehog signaling pathway

KEY POINTS

- The main cause of squamous and basal skin cancer is exposure to ultraviolet (UV) radiation.
- Ultraviolet radiation, consistent of a small UV-B and complete UV-A band, is responsible for the biological effects on human skin.
- Destruction of repair mechanisms or activation of oncogenes may lead to carcinogenesis. Pathways involving p53, tumor supressor gene, apoptosis, transforming growth factor β, platelet-derivated growth factor, telomerase enzyme and hedgehog signaling system may participate in this process.
- Better understanding and increased awareness of molecular mechanisms underlying nonmelanoma skin cancer may aid in development of innovative diagnostic, therapeutic, and preventive measures.

INTRODUCTION

Cancer is a cellular disease characterized by a transformed cell population with abnormal cell growth. Malignant transformation is an irreversible transition of one cell that leads to the formation of a cancer. Histopathologic examination is the gold standard for the diagnosis of skin cancer. In the future, analysis of molecular parameters such as nucleic acids and DNA will also gain importance for diagnosis, prognosis, and therapy.[1] Understanding the molecular mechanisms underlying the pathogenesis of nonmelanoma skin cancer of the head and neck of growing importance for the diagnostician and surgeon alike.

ULTRAVIOLET RADIATION

The main cause of skin cancer is exposure to ultraviolet (UV) radiation. The solar UV spectrum consists of UVC (wavelengths below 280 nm), UVB (280–315 nm), and UVA bands (315–400 nm). The predominant part of the short-wave, high-energy, and destructive UV spectrum cannot reach the Earth's surface: the ozone layer in the outer Earth atmosphere absorbs the shorter wavelengths up to 310 nm (UVC and main part of UVB radiation). The remaining transmitted UV spectrum, that is, a small UVB and the complete UVA band, is responsible for biological effects on human skin.[2]

[a] Department of Otorhinolaryngology, Kanuni Education and Research Hospital, Trabzon, Turkey; [b] Department of Otolaryngology, New York University Langone Medical Center, NY, USA; [c] Department of Otolaryngology, Faculty of Medicine, Karadeniz Technical University, Trabzon, Turkey 61200
* Corresponding author.
E-mail address: benguyc@yahoo.com

Facial Plast Surg Clin N Am 20 (2012) 437–443
http://dx.doi.org/10.1016/j.fsc.2012.07.006

The consistently increasing incidence of melanocytic and nonmelanocytic skin tumors is associated with recreational sun exposure. Epidemiologic data indicate that excessive or cumulative sunlight exposure takes place years before the cancer occurs. The most important protection strategies against UV damage in human skin consist of melanin synthesis and active DNA-repair mechanisms. DNA is the major target of direct and indirect UV damage.[1]

Animal models have demonstrated that UVB is more likely than UVA to induce skin cancer. UV-induced DNA photoproducts are able to cause specific mutations (UV-signature) in susceptible genes for squamous cell carcinoma (SCC) and basal cell carcinoma (BCC). In SCC, development of UV-signature mutations in the p53 tumor suppressor gene are the most common event, as precancerous lesions reveal fewer than 80% and SCCs more than 90% UV-specific p53 mutations.[3]

UV light does not penetrate the body any deeper than the skin and is absorbed by the different skin layers in a wavelength-dependent manner. UVB is almost completely absorbed by the epidermis; only 10% to 20% of UVB energy reaches the epidermal stratum basale and papillary dermis. UVA penetrates deeper into the dermis and deposits 30% to 50% of its energy into the papillary dermis. These absorption characteristics of human skin explain why UVB effects occur predominantly in the epidermis (development of skin cancer) whereas UVA effects occur in the dermis (solar elastosis, skin aging). UV radiation also displays immunosuppressive effects and is able to generate tolerance against immunogenetic skin tumors. Thus UV is considered to be a "double-edged sword," causing skin cancer by DNA damage on the one hand and enabling tumor escape from immune surveillance on the other.[2]

UV-INDUCED CARCINOGENESIS IN SQUAMOUS CELL CARCINOMA

The precursor cell of SCC and its precancerous progenitor, the actinic keratosis (AK), is assumed to be the interfollicular epidermal basal keratinocyte. AK and SCC are strongly related to UV exposure because 90% occur at predilection sites where the skin is regularly exposed to sun damage:

- Head
- Forehead
- Nose
- Ears
- Back of hands

The lifetime risk of developing an SCC correlates very closely with the individual cumulative UV dose.[4] De Gruijl[3] demonstrated a wavelength dependency of SCC induction effectiveness by means of hairless mice. SCC were generated in AK by UV with UV-action spectrum peaks at 300 nm in the UVB band that continuously decreased through the UVA band, with a smaller peak at 380 nm. Similar findings were observed in the murine model. When these findings were applied to estimates of human skin tolerance, the relative efficacy to induce SCC at 300 nm UVB irradiation was 1000-fold higher than UVA.[5]

UVA predominantly causes photosensitizer-mediated oxidative DNA damage. Because in this part of the UVA spectrum (347–400 nm) direct DNA damage is not observed, it can be assumed that the indirect oxidative UVA effects contribute to the mutagenic potential of UVA in this wavelength range. UVB is even more powerful than UVA in its ability to induce AK and SCC, and is considered to be the predominant carcinogen.[2]

The most important protein involved in early UV-induced carcinogenesis of SCC appears to be the tumor suppressor p53. p53 is an essential and well-defined transcription factor regulating cell-cycle control and apoptosis.[6] UV radiation helps to stabilize transcriptional activity and protein degradation. Specific p53 mutations can be found in 75% to 80% of AK and in more than 90% of cutaneous SCC.[7]

UV-INDUCED CARCINOGENESIS IN BASAL CELL CARCINOMA

BCC is the most common malignancy in Caucasians, with a worldwide increasing incidence. Exposure to UV radiation is assumed to be the main causative pathogenic factor for BCCs as well, but the precise relation between amount, timing, and pattern of UV exposure and BCC risk is still unknown. Compared with SCC, the correlation of UV with basal cell carcinogenesis is far less obvious, and epidemiologic data are not completely in line with the impact of cumulative UV dose. Some studies reveal a link between cumulative UV dose and BCC risk, although the relative risks are small, with odds ratios of 1.0 to 1.5.[8]

BCCs predominantly affect[9]:

- Seborrheic central parts of the face: root of nose, nasal ala, nasolabial fold
- Head
- Trunk
- Lower limbs

The BCC precursor cell is less well defined than that of SCC and is hypothesized to stem from interfollicular epidermal basal keratinocytes with retained basal morphology, from the follicular outer root sheath or sebaceous gland derived keratinocytes. The deeper anatomic localization of the BCC cells originating in hair follicles and sebaceous glands may be one explanation for differences in the carcinogenesis of BCC and SCC.[2]

BCCs are predominantly sporadic but also appear in persons suffering from rare hereditary disorders such as nevoid BCC syndrome (NBCCS; Gorlin syndrome) or xeroderma pigmentosum (XP).

The most common inherited disorder associated with BCCs is NBCCS. NBCCS is an autosomal dominant neurocutaneous disorder. Affected individuals have a wide range of developmental anomalies, including skeletal abnormalities, craniofacial dysmorphism, and macrocephaly. Multiple early-onset BCCs are a hallmark of the syndrome that also includes features such as odontogenic keratocysts, palmar and plantar pits, and calcification of the falx cerebri. In addition to BCCs, patients have an increased incidence of medulloblastomas, meningiomas, and ovarian and cardiac fibromas. Germline mutations in the PTCH (patched) gene are found in the majority of patients with this syndrome.[10]

XP is caused by inherited defects in nucleotide excision repair (NER) genes, resulting in a complex skin pathology including lentigines, epidermal hyperplasias, BCCs, SCCs, and cutaneous melanomas triggered by exposure to the sun. This disease is an exaggerated response to UV light, with the early onset of a vastly increased number of skin lesions that would otherwise occur in small numbers late in life. Because of the deficient DNA repair, the rate at which skin cancers develop in young XP patients is increased at least 1000-fold.[1]

THE HEDGEHOG SIGNALING PATHWAY

The hedgehog pathway is a fundamental signal transduction pathway in embryogenesis that is responsible for the proper development of various organs, including:

- Neural tube
- Axial skeleton
- Limbs
- Lungs
- Teeth
- Skin
- Hair

Consequently, germline mutations in genes encoding members of the hedgehog pathway result in human diseases characterized by tumor predisposition and/or developmental defects.[11]

The Hh gene, encoding a secret ligand, was originally identified in screens for mutations that disrupt segment polarity in the fruit-fly *Drosophila*. The gene has 3 vertebrate homologues, of which sonic Hh (Shh) is the most widely expressed. The Hh ligand binds to the membrane receptor PTCH1. On binding, PTCH1-mediated inhibition of the transmembrane protein, smoothened (SMOH), is relieved, allowing the latter to transduce a signal into the cell. This process results in altered activity of the Gli family of transcription factors. In fact, the binding of Hh to PTCH1 switches on Gli-mediated expression of pathway target genes such as PTCH1 and Gli1.[12]

In the absence of hedgehog, Ptc inhibits signal transduction by repressing SMOH activity. Binding of hedgehog to Ptc abrogates Ptc-mediated inhibition of SMOH, and the signal is transduced from the cytoplasm into the nucleus via a large, microtubulin-associated protein complex. Although vertebrate homologues have been identified for most of the *Drosophila* hedgehog pathway genes, the vertebrate pathway seems to be more complex and is far less well understood. There are 3 different hedgehog proteins identified in vertebrates[13]:

1. Desert hedgehog (Dhh)
2. Indian hedgehog (Ihh)
3. Sonic hedgehog (Shh)

The most striking evidence that Hh pathway deregulation is an early event in BCC formation comes from in vivo transgenic model systems. In these studies the Hh pathway was deregulated in both epidermal cells of transgenic mice and transgenic, reconstituted human skin. Tumors that were indistinguishable from BCC developed within weeks, in the absence of mutation in other genes such as HRAS and TP53. Based on these studies, current evidence shows that Hh pathway deregulation alone can rapidly generate BCC directly from normal keratinocytes. This finding may explain why, in contrast to melanoma and SCC, BCC has no apparent precursor lesion.[13]

P53 TUMOR SUPPRESSOR GENE

The p53 tumor suppressor gene was first described in 1979 and was initially classified as an oncogene because of its ability to transform cells.[14] As a consequence of exposure to sunlight, about 70% of nonmelanoma skin cancers (NMSC) are induced by UV radiation. To counteract carcinogenic effects of UV, epidermal cells activate mechanisms that control cell proliferation, DNA repair, and apoptosis. Activation of p53 tumor suppressor protein occurs in response to a variety of cellular stresses including DNA damage, oncogenic stimulation, hypoxia, oxidative stress, or telomere shortening, and directs cells toward cell-cycle arrest or apoptosis depending on the amount of DNA damage. This process allows p53 to exert its function as a "guardian of the genome" and tumor suppressor by blocking proliferative expansion of damaged cells.[15]

p53 DNA Repair

p53-Induced GI arrest allows the cellular repair pathways to remove possible DNA lesions before the onset of DNA synthesis and mitosis, whereas p53-induced apoptosis eliminates potential progenitors of malignant tumor cells. p53 participates in DNA repair by activating the GI/S cell-cycle check point and allowing more time for DNA repair, and also by inducing transcriptional activation of at least several known genes directly participating in DNA repair. With NER, p53 transactivates 2 xeroderma pigmentosum–associated gene products, p48XPE and XPC, which are involved in recognition of DNA damage. A third p53-regulated protein is GADD45, which binds to UV-damaged DNA in vitro. p53 also participates in base excision repair (BER) by regulating DNA polymerase p, which is directly involved in DNA-repair synthesis.[16]

p53 Mutations

p53 is a key regulatory molecule in the cellular response to UV radiation, and the TP53 mutation is the most common alteration in nonmelanoma skin cancer. The MDM2 oncogene negatively regulates p53 protein levels, and both genes have functional polymorphisms that may modify the risk for skin cancer. Furthermore, prior research suggests that TP53 mutations preferentially occur on the arginine allele to selectively inactivate the p63 pathway. Recent research on susceptibility and preferential mutation in nonmelanoma skin cancer showed that The TP53 Arg72Pro and MDM2 309 polymorphisms were genotyped in a population-based case-control study of nonmelanoma skin cancer, and TP53 alteration (mutation and immunohistochemistry staining) was also evaluated. There was an association between TP53 alterations in the tumors and constitutive TP53 genotype, with alterations preferentially occurring on the proline allele.[1]

Analysis of mutations in p53 gene has established an unequivocal connection between UV exposure, DNA damage, and skin carcinogenesis. UVB and UVC radiation induces unique types of DNA damage, producing cyclobutane-type pyrimidine dimers (CPD) and pyrimidine (G-A) or (6-4 t)

pyrimidone photoproducts. These unique lesions in the DNA give rise to unique mutations. UV radiation induces predominantly C→T and CC→TT transitions at dipyrimidine sequences, which have become the "signature" of UV-induced mutagenesis.[16]

Many researchers studied gene mutations in a large proportion of human SCCs and BCCs. Brash and colleagues[17] revealed p53 mutation in 58% of human SCCs. Rady and colleagues[18] have demonstrated p53 mutations in human BCCs at 50% frequency. Bolshakov and colleagues[19] analyzed 342 tissues from patients with aggressive and nonaggressive BCCs and SCCs for p53 mutations by single-strand conformation polymorphism and nucleotide sequencing. p53 mutations were detected in 33 of 50 aggressive BCCs (66%), 37 of 98 nonaggressive BCCs (38%), 28 of 80 aggressive SCCs (35%), 28 of 56 nonaggressive SCCs (50%), and 3 of 29 samples of sun-exposed skin (10%). About 71% of the p53 mutations detected in aggressive and nonaggressive BCCs and SCCs were UV-signature mutations.

In addition, Ziegler and colleagues[20] found that 45% of human BCCs contained a second point mutation on the other p53 allele. Stern and colleagues[21] have also analyzed nonmelanoma skin tumors from psoriasis patients treated with psoralen + UVA. In 69 tumors, 37 (54%) tumors had 1 or more p53 mutations, of which 17 (46%) tumors had only UV-type mutations, 2 (5%) tumors had only psoralen + UVA–type mutations, and 18 (49%) tumors had both types of mutations. p53 mutations have also been found at high frequencies in skin cancers from patients with base substitutions of the genetic disorder XP. In a study of skin cancers from XP patients, Dumaz and colleagues[22] showed that p53 mutations were present in 17 of 43 (40%) patients and that 61% of these mutations were tandem CC→TT base substitutions.

Immunosuppressed patients of renal allografts (RAR) are also at much higher risk for the development of skin cancer. Overexpression of p53 protein and p53 mutations has been detected in a large proportion of SCCs and premalignant lesions in RAR patients. Cairey-Remonnay and colleagues[23] analyzed 53 SCCs from 40 kidney-transplant recipients. The rate of arginine homozygosity in SCC in renal transplant patients was significantly higher (83%) than in immunocompetent patients with or without SCC (60% and 59%, respectively). The TP53 arginine/arginine genotype may represent a potential risk factor for the development of SCC in kidney-transplant recipients in comparison with immunocompetent patients.

APOPTOSIS

A major feature of NMSC cells is their resistance to programmed cell death or apoptosis. The reason for this is not entirely clear. The extrinsic caspase-8–dependent apoptotic pathway is mediated by death-ligands and their receptors of the tumor necrosis factor (TNF) and TNF-receptor (TNF-R) family. For example, Fas-ligand (FasL) or TRAIL (TNF-related apoptosis–inducing ligand) induce caspase-dependent apoptosis of cells on interaction with their corresponding receptors, Fas or TRAIL-receptors (TRAIL-Rs).[24]

The apoptotic process can be modulated by several regulatory proteins such as caspase inhibitors and other apoptosis inhibitors, including decoy receptors, cellular Flice inhibitory protein (FLIP), and survivin. The intrinsic apoptotic pathway is mainly mitochondria dependent. It is extensively used in response to internal insults such as DNA damage. This pathway is executed by the members of the bcl-2 family. Different members of the bcl-2 family can function in opposite ways. Most cancer cells exhibit defective apoptotic mechanisms or develop mechanisms to evade apoptosis, allowing them to develop in an uncontrolled way. Therefore, restoring apoptosis is a promising way to treat cancers.[25]

The formation of NMSC is a consequence of long-term UV exposure of the skin. If UV-damaged DNA cannot be repaired or the DNA-damaged cell is not eliminated by apoptosis cell transformation, tumor development can be the outcome.

FasL, a member of the tumor necrosis superfamily, is a key molecule involved in the elimination of sunburn cells. FasL is expressed in normal skin epidermis, preferentially in the basal layer. Regulation of FasL expression has a dual effect on cancerogenesis. On the other hand, once a BCC or SCC has developed, FasL is strongly upregulated. High expression of FasL may now serve to protect the tumor from the attack of immune effector cells.

If DNA repair is not possible, the DNA-damaged keratinocytes are eliminated by apoptosis (sunburn cells) under the control of the *p53* gene. It has been shown that FasL is central for the formation of sunburn cells. Certain individuals have a lower DNA-repair capacity, and thus a higher risk not only of developing skin cancers but also of having a greater number of skin cancers. A good example is the XP patient. However, the *p53* gene can itself be a direct target of UV radiation. If mutations occur in this gene, this can lead to uncontrolled cell proliferation and loss of apoptosis in these cells. As a consequence, BCCs or SCCs may develop. Mutations in the *p53* gene are detected in 56% of BCCs and in more than 90% of SCCs.[26]

TRANSFORMING GROWTH FACTOR β PATHWAY OF NONMELANOMA SKIN CANCER

Since its discovery in 1981, transforming growth factor (TGF)-β has been recognized as a potent inhibitor of epithelial cell growth.[27] Some carcinoma cell lines escape from TGF-β growth inhibition and display a direct role of TGF-β as an autocrine stimulator of tumor-cell invasion and metastasis. In the past decade, a large quantity of experimental evidence has accumulated suggesting a dual role for TGF-β in cancer. It is now widely accepted that TGF-β can act as a tumor suppressor at early stages of tumorigenesis and as a potent driver of malignant progression, invasion, and metastasis at later stages.[28] The expression of TGF-β is regulated by the hedgehog signaling pathway. In adult tissues, TGF-β proteins are dynamically expressed in hair follicles and have been implicated in the cyclic growth of hair, including the remodeling of extracellular matrix. Studies show that a potential growth inhibitory escape mechanism exists for BCCs by downregulating TGF-β in tumor cells. The results also suggest a possible role for TGF-β signaling in stromal cells that could contribute to local tumor invasion. However, the evidence to date for an involvement of TGF-β signaling in the development of BCCs is merely circumstantial.[29]

PLATELET-DERIVED GROWTH FACTOR

Platelet-derived growth factor (PDGF) isoforms are important mitogens for different types of mesenchymal cells, which have important functions during embryonal development and in the adult during wound healing and tissue homeostasis. In tumors, PDGF isoforms are often overexpressed, and contribute to the growth of both normal and malignant cells.

PDGF expression has been demonstrated in several different solid tumors, from glioblastomas to prostate carcinomas. In recent years the role of PDGF in the proliferation of nonmelanoma skin cancers has been established. Dermatofibrosarcoma protuberans (DFSP) and giant-cell fibroblastoma (GCF) are recurrent, infiltrative skin tumors of intermediate malignancy. The autocrine growth stimulation of tumor cells by PDGF is well demonstrated in many types of tumors including DFSP and BCCs of the skin.[30] In addition, PDGF can regulate stromal cells through a paracrine mechanism that is observed in skin SCCs and melanomas. Improved methods for detection of activated PDGF receptors would be most useful for screens of PDGF-signaling–activated tumors.

Discovering the importance of PDGF signaling for the development of BCCs not only provides a molecular basis of hedgehog-signaling–mediated tumorigenesis, but also has significant therapeutic implications such as interferon-α treatment and inhibition of PDGF signaling, in addition to cryosurgery and suppression of the Shh pathway for BCC treatments. Additional research on PDGF signaling in other cutaneous malignancies will certainly help in the design of better ways to treat these cancers.[31]

TELOMERASE

Telomerase, a ribonucleoprotein, is capable of adding telomeric sequences (TTAGGG hexameric repeats) to the ends of chromosomes and thereby halting the erosion of the chromosome at each cell division. The most important function of telomerase consists in elongating the tandemly repeated TTAGGG-DNA sequences of the chromosome ends (telomere; tele = end). In the absence of telomerase, telomere DNA is lost after each successive cell division.[32] This process leads to the progressive shortening of the telomeres because the DNA polymerase of eukaryotic cells is not able to completely copy the DNA at the ends of linear chromosomes. This phenomenon is known as the end replication problem. Whereas most normal somatic cells contain minimal or no detectable telomerase activity, most immortal and tumor cells exhibit significant levels of telomerase activity and show no loss of telomere length during proliferation. The evaluation of telomerase has been proposed for diagnostic and therapeutic purposes in human cancer. The precise molecular events in skin carcinogenesis are numerous, complicated, and not yet completely understood. In a recent study telomerase was evaluated in 35 BCCs and 14 SCCs. A higher telomerase messenger level was shown to be associated with SCCs, as was a higher telomerase activity. The role of telomerase in skin cancer may be elucidated using reverse transcription–polymerase chain reaction for telomerase RNA. As a tool this is easier and faster than the TRAP (telomeric repeat amplification protocol) assay in identifying more aggressive malignancies among nonmelanoma skin specimens.[32]

The activation of telomerase plays an important role in the cancerogenesis of cutaneous BCCs and SCCs as well as in oral SCCs. This role is implied by the simultaneous appearance of telomerase with UV exposure in normal skin. In most studies, telomerase is more activated in BCC than in SCC, which can be explained by the high proliferation rate of BCC. Telomerase activation in BCC and SCC of the head and neck region is more likely a proliferation marker than a prognostic marker. Activation of telomerase in the immediate tumor-free margin of BCC points to the emergence of field cancerization because the interval without relapse is shorter in these patients. It is conceivable that the relapse rate in patients with a telomerase-positive tumor-free margin can be reduced with adjuvant antitelomerase therapy. Studies have shown that telomerase activation in SCC margins is an immune response associated with a longer interval without recurrence, so that adjuvant antitelomerase therapy may be contraindicated for these patients.[33]

Killian and colleagues found that the telomere lengths significantly differ between BCC in renal transplant patients and normal populations, and between BCC and SCC in these same patient groups.[34] In this study the telomere-length dynamics are markedly different between BCC and SCC. These findings increase our understanding of the differing biological properties of these NMSC tumors, and also may clarify the differences in the incidence rates between BCC and SCC in immunocompromised patients. It is highly likely that future treatments of these cancers that involve targeting of telomere-maintenance mechanisms will have different outcomes for BCC and SCC, including those in the renal transplant population. It will therefore be important to further clarify the differences between the telomere-maintenance pathways in these cancers.[34]

SUMMARY

Molecular mechanisms play important roles in understanding the pathogenesis of nonmelanoma skin cancers of the head and neck. Increased awareness of these molecular changes may aid in the development of new diagnostic, therapeutic, and preventive measures.

REFERENCES

1. Ponten F, Lundeberg J, Asplund A. Principles of tumor biology and pathogenesis of BCCs and SCCs. In: Bolognia JL, Jorizzo JL, Rapini RP, editors. Dermatology, 2nd edition. St Louis (MO): Mosby; 2008:1635–7, 1651–2.
2. Rass K. UV damage and DNA repair in basal cell and squamous cell carcinomas. In: Reichrath J, editor. Molecular mechanisms of basal cell and squamous cell carcinomas. New York: Springer; 2006. p. 18–22.
3. De Gruijl FR. Skin cancer and solar UV radiation. Eur J Cancer 1999;35:2003–9.
4. Vitasa BC, Taylor HR, Strickland PJ, et al. Association of nonmelanoma skin cancer and actinic

keratosis with cumulative solar ultraviolet exposure in Maryland watermen. Cancer 1990;65:2811–7.

5. De Gruijl FR, Sterenborg HJ, Forbes PD, et al. Wavelength dependence of skin cancer induction by ultraviolet irradiation of albino hairless mice. Cancer Res 1993;53:53–60.

6. Vogelstein B, Kinzler KW. P53 function and dysfunction. Cell 1992;70:523–6.

7. Brash DE, Ziegler A, Jonason AS, et al. Sunlight and sunburn in human skin cancer: p53, apoptosis and tumor promotion. J Investig Dermatol Symp Proc 1996;1:136–42.

8. Zanetti R, Rosso S, Martinez C, et al. The multicentre South European study 'Helios': skin characteristics and sunburn in basal cell and squamous carcinomas of the skin. Br J Cancer 1996;73:1447–54.

9. Corona R, Dogliotti E, D'Ericco M, et al. Risk factors for basal cell carcinoma in a Mediterranean population. Arch Dermatol 2002;137:1162–8.

10. Gorlin RJ. Nevoid basal cell carcinoma syndrome. Medicine 1987;66:98–113.

11. Peacock CD, Rudin CM. Skin deep and deeper: multiple pathways in basal cell carcinogenesis. Cancer Prev Res (Phila) 2010;3(10):1213–6.

12. Saldanha G, Fletcher A, Slater DN. Basal cell carcinoma: a dermatopathological and molecular biological update. Br J Dermatol 2003;148:195–202.

13. Reifenberger J. The hedgehog signaling pathway and epithelial skin cancer. In: Reichrath J, editor. Molecular mechanisms of basal cell and squamous cell carcinomas. New York: Landes Bioscience and Springer Science; 2006. p. 58–61.

14. Levine AJ. P53, the cellular gatekeeper for growth and division. Cell 1997;88:321–31.

15. Lane DP. P53, guardian of the genome. Nature 1992; 358:15–6.

16. Melnikova VO, Ananthaswamy HN. P53 Protein and nonmelanoma skin cancer. In: Reichrath J, editor. Molecular mechanisms of basal cell and squamous cell carcinomas. New York: Landes Bioscience and Springer Science; 2006. p. 66–71.

17. Brash DE, Rudolph JA, Simon JA, et al. A role for sunlight in skin cancer: UV induced p53 mutations in squamous cell carcinoma. Proc Natl Acad Sci U S A 1991;88:10124–8.

18. Rady P, Scinicariello F, Wagner RF, et al. p53 mutations in basal cell carcinomas. Cancer Res 1992;52:3804–6.

19. Bolshakov S, Walker CM, Strom SS, et al. p53 mutations in human aggressive and nonaggressive basal and squamous cell carcinomas. Clin Cancer Res 2003;9:228–34.

20. Ziegler A, Jonason AS, Leffell DJ, et al. Sunburn and p53 in the onset of skin cancer. Nature 1994;372: 773–6.

21. Stern RS, Bolshakov S, Nataraj AJ, et al. p53 mutation in nonmelanoma skin cancers occurring in psoralen ultraviolet a-treated patients: evidence for heterogeneity and field cancerization. J Invest Dermatol 2002;119:522–6.

22. Dumaz N, Drougard C, Sarasin A, et al. Specific UV-induced mutation spectrum in the p53 gene of skin tumors in DNA repair deficient xeroderma pigmentosum patients. Proc Natl Acad Sci U S A 1993;90:10529–33.

23. Cairey-Remonnay S, Humbey O, Mougin C, et al. TP53 polymorphism of exon 4 at codon 72 in cutaneous squamous cell carcinoma and benign epithelial lesions of renal transplant recipients and immunocompetent individuals: lack of correlation with human papillomavirus status. J Invest Dermatol 2002;118(6):1026–31.

24. Erb P, Ji J, Wernli M, et al. Role of apoptosis in basal cell and squamous cell carcinoma formation. Immunol Lett 2005;100:68–72.

25. Li HL, Zhu H, Xu CJ, et al. Cleavage of BID by caspase 8 mediates the mitochondrial damage in the Fas pathway of apoptosis. Cell 1998;94:491–501.

26. Erb P, Ji J, Wernli M, et al. Apoptosis and cancerogenesis of basal cell and squamous cell carcinoma. In: Reichrath J, editor. Molecular mechanisms of basal cell and squamous cell carcinomas. New York: Landes Bioscience and Springer Science; 2006. p. 108–12.

27. Moses HL, Branum EB, Proper JA, et al. Transforming growth factor production by chemically transformed cells. Cancer Res 1981;41:2842–8.

28. Derynck R, Akhurst RJ, Balmain A. TGF-β signaling in tumor suppression and cancer progression. Nat Genet 2001;29:117–29.

29. Quintanilla M, Perez-Gomez E, Romero D, et al. TGF-β pathway and cancerogenesis of epithelial skin tumors. In: Reichrath J, editor. Molecular mechanisms of basal cell and squamous cell carcinomas. New York: Landes Bioscience and Springer Science; 2006. p. 80–7.

30. Heldin CH. Autocrine PDGF stimulation in malignancies. Ups J Med Sci 2012;117:83–91.

31. Xie J. PDGF pathways and growth of basal cell and squamous cell carcinomas. In: Reichrath J, editor. Molecular mechanisms of basal cell and squamous cell carcinomas. New York: Landes Bioscience and Springer Science; 2006. p. 94–100.

32. Boldrini L, Loggini B, Gisfredi S, et al. Evaluation of telomerase in non-melanoma skin cancer. Int J Mol Med 2003;11(5):607–11.

33. Fabricius EM. The role of telomerase for cancerogenesis of basal cell and squamous cell carcinomas. In: Reichrath J, editor. Molecular mechanisms of basal cell and squamous cell carcinomas. New York: Landes Bioscience and Springer Science; 2006. p. 115–20.

34. Killian P, Lynch A, al Nooh F, et al. The different telomere lengths in basal and squamous cell carcinomas also differ between the nontransplant and renal transplant population. Hum Pathol 2008;39:1034–104.

Nonmelanoma Skin Cancer of the Head and Neck
Nonsurgical Treatment

Aylin Türel Ermertcan, MD[a],*, Peter W. Hellings, MD[b],
Cemal Cingi, MD[c]

KEYWORDS

- Skin cancer • Nonmelanoma • Treatment • Nonsurgical

KEY POINTS

- Alternatives to the surgical management for nonmelanoma skin cancer may be preferred under certain circumstances:
  - Tumors that are multifocal, extensive, in cosmetically sensitive areas, or not amenable to simple surgical treatment
  - Areas that may result in significant scarring after surgical intervention
  - Older people with more surgical risk factors
- Cryotherapy, curettage and electrodesiccation, radiation therapy, photodynamic therapy, laser, interferon, imiquimod, retinoids, and 5-fluorouracil have been demonstrated to be effective for the treatment of NMSC.

INTRODUCTION

Nonmelanoma skin cancer (NMSC) is one of the most common types of cancer in the world; the two most prevalent forms are basal cell carcinoma (BCC) and squamous cell carcinoma (SCC). Epidemiologic studies investigating the prevalence of NMSC in the general population indicate that the number of cases has increased rapidly over the last 2 decades.[1] The incidence of NMSCs was estimated at 1.3 million cases for the year 2000 and is increasing.[2,3] More than 1 000 000 new cases and 1000 deaths were reported in the United States in 2009.[4–6] BCC is the most common skin cancer and composes 75% of NMSC. SCC is the second most common skin cancer, accounting for 20% of cases of NMSC.[2,7] Although the relative mortality is low (0.1%), NMSCs may cause considerable morbidity, particularly in visible areas, such as the head and neck, with consequent unacceptable cosmetic outcomes and/or functional impairments, causing direct and indirect costs of management in the order of billions of dollars annually.[4–6,8]

The goal of NMSC treatment is complete eradication of the tumor with preservation of the surrounding structures in an aesthetically acceptable manner. Several treatment options, both surgical and nonsurgical, are available. Mohs micrographic surgery is the therapeutic gold standard for all NMSCs in terms of cure rates, margin control, and tissue conservation.[2,3] However, surgical removal can also cause significant disfigurement and functional impairment. Alternatives to the surgical management may be preferred under certain circumstances. Some tumors may be multifocal, extensive, in cosmetically sensitive areas, or not amenable to simple surgical treatment. Significant scarring may result after surgical intervention, depending on the location of the lesion, as in the

[a] Department of Dermatology, Faculty of Medicine, Celal Bayar University, Manisa 45010, Turkey; [b] Department of Otorhinolaryngology, University Hospitals, Leuven, Belgium; [c] Department of Otorhinolaryngology, Faculty of Medicine, Eskisehir Osmangazi University, Eskişehir, Turkey
* Corresponding author.
E-mail address: draylinturel@hotmail.com

Facial Plast Surg Clin N Am 20 (2012) 445–454
http://dx.doi.org/10.1016/j.fsc.2012.08.004
1064-7406/12/$ – see front matter © 2012 Elsevier Inc. All rights reserved.

case of small superficial BCCs on the shoulders and central chest, which may produce hypertrophic scarring or spread scarring disproportionate to the initial size of the lesion. In addition, as the population of older people, who may have more surgical risk factors, continues to increase, a careful assessment of surgical risk factors will need to be taken into account both preoperatively and perioperatively for an increasing proportion of patients.[2] Skin cancer incidence increases with age, as do other medical problems; a nonsurgical option may be a strong consideration as an alternative treatment choice.[2,9]

Cryotherapy, curettage and electrodesiccation, radiation therapy, photodynamic therapy, laser, interferon (IFN), imiquimod, retinoids, and 5-fluorouracil (5-FU) have been demonstrated to be effective for the treatment of NMSC.[1,4,10–16]

This review article explores the available nonsurgical treatment options, their indications, and their efficacy (**Table 1**).

CRYOTHERAPY

Cryotherapy involves tissue destruction by application of extreme cold to the lesion using liquid nitrogen. Vaporizing liquid nitrogen is brought into contact with the skin lesion to freeze it. This approach destroys superficial tissue. Cryotherapy is a simple, rapid, and inexpensive method (**Fig. 1**). The optimum duration of freezing is not known, but the lowest rates of recurrence are obtained using aggressive protocols. Several cryotherapy sessions may be needed.[14] Because not all cells die after the first freeze-thaw cycle, treatment is generally repeated. Tumor cells are known to be very sensitive to cryosurgery because of their high content of water, higher metabolism, and microcirculation. Connective tissue is less sensitive, whereas fibroblasts are relatively resistant to cold.[17] This modality has been recommended for the treatment of actinic keratosis (AK), Bowen disease (BD), superficial BCC, small nodular BCC, and small well-differentiated SCC.[18]

The practical requirements for effective cell killing by cryosurgery are rapid freezing at a rate greater than $100°C/min$, tissue temperature less than $-25°C$, slow thawing at a rate of $10°C/min$ or less, and at least 2 freeze-thaw cycles. BCCs require 2×40 to 60 seconds, this time must be adjusted depending on the size and depth of the tumor and on individual differences; sometimes a third freeze-thaw cycle is needed. The cryotherapy of cutaneous malignancies is considered to be an alternative method because surgical excision provides histologic control and a more rapidly healing wound.[17] Cryosurgical treatment of BCCs gives cure rates that compare favorably with other

modes of therapy provided the correct technique is used and the treatment is limited to small (<20 mm), well-defined, previously untreated tumors, avoiding BCCs on the inner canthus of the eye, nasolabial and retro-auricular folds, and the hair-bearing scalp.[19–21] Some investigators advocate debulking the tumor using curettage or electrosurgery before cryotherapy.[19,22] The recommended temperature is between $-50°C$ and $-60°C$ at the base of the tumor, and the freeze time is approximately 45 seconds for a 1-cm lesion. During the past 2 decades, there has been an increased use of colder temperatures. There are some contraindications for cryosurgery. Patients who have cold urticaria, cold intolerance, cryofibrinogenemia, or cryoglobulinemia are best treated by other means. Tumors with indistinct or ill-defined borders (eg, morpheaform or infiltrative histologic subtypes) as well as deeply penetrating and very aggressive lesions are best treated by other modalities. Some anatomic areas where cryosurgery should be undertaken cautiously include the corners of the mouth, the vermilion margin of the lips, eyebrows, inner canthi, the free margin of the ala nasi, and the auditory canal because scarring or retraction of the tissue can occur.[23]

Although hypopigmentation is a frequent consequence of cryosurgery for skin tumors, wounds tend to heal without significant tissue contraction, and this can give rise to excellent cosmetic results for some patients.[18] Occasionally, hypertrophic scarring may develop, particularly after treatment of a large lesion; but this always improves and resolves with time, usually within months.[23]

In the literature, it has been reported that the 5-year cure rate is 97% to 99% for nonmelanoma skin cancers.[20,21,23] Zacarian[24] reported an 18-year cure rate of 97.4% in the treatment of 4228 carcinomas.

CURETTAGE AND ELECTRODESICCATION

Electrodesiccation and electrofulguration represent the most commonly uses of electrosurgery in dermatology. Although often used to denote the same procedure, there is a subtle technical difference between the two. With electrodesiccation, the electrode tip is in contact with the tissue; with electrofulguration, there is a 1- to 2-mm separation (**Fig. 2**). Electrodesiccation or fulguration is commonly used in the treatment of BCCs and SCCs less than 2 cm in diameter. When treating selected BCCs and SCCs, curettage must be followed by electrodesiccation. The bulk of the tumor should be removed by vigorous curettage followed by light electrodesiccation of the base of the lesion with a 2- to 3-mm margin of surrounding skin.[25]

Table 1
Summary of nonsurgical treatment of NMSC of the head and neck

Treatment	Indications	Drawbacks
Cryotherapy	Previously untreated superficial BCCs, small nodular BCCs, and small well-differentiated SCCs	Tumors with indistinct or ill-defined borders, deeply penetrating and aggressive lesions Some anatomic areas, such as the corners of the mouth, the vermilion margin of the lips, eyebrows, inner canthi, the free margin of the ala nasi, and the auditory canal Cold urticaria, cold intolerance, cryofibrinogenemia, or cryoglobulinemia
Curettage and electrodesiccation	BCCs <2 cm in diameter Small SCCs in situ and well-differentiated primary SCCs <1 cm in diameter	Central facial BCCs and infiltrating, micronodular, or morphealike histologic type Larger and higher-risk SCCs
Photodynamic therapy	BCCs, especially multiple lesions In situ SCCs	Invasive SCCs Generalized photosensitivity, facial edema, and pain
Radiotherapy	Patients older than 60 y for small primary SCCs at sites other than hands, feet, or genital organs Adjuvant to Mohs surgery in the event of extensive perineural invasion In addition to incomplete excision of low-risk SCCs After primary surgery, if the margins are ambiguous and further surgery is thought not to be appropriate	Verrucous SCCs BCCs recurred after previous radiotherapy The morpheic BCC subtype or the presence of underlying bone or cartilage involvement
Lasers	Superficial BCCs	Invasive BCCs and SCCs
Topical 5-fluorouracil	Superficial BCCs and selected SCCs in situ	Invasive BCCs and SCCs
Imiquimod	Superficial BCCs and SCCs in situ mostly in patients in whom surgery is not an option	Invasive BCCs and SCCs
Retinoids	Prevention of new BCCs and SCCs	—
Cytokines	BCCs Debulking large tumors Treatment of positive margins after surgical excision	—
Cyclooxygenase-2 inhibitors	Prevention of new BCCs and SCCs	—
Cyclopamine	BCC	—
GDC-0449 (vismodegib)	BCC	—
Epidermal growth factor inhibitors	SCC	—
Afamelanotide	SCC	—
Capecitabine	Prevention of recurrences	—

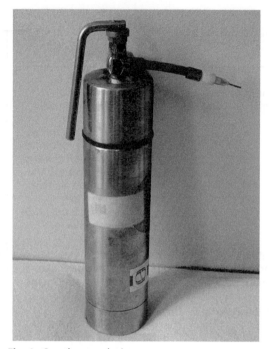

Fig. 1. Cryotherapy device.

This modality can be used for the same spectrum of lesions as cryotherapy.[18]

The large, multiple superficial BCCs found on the trunk are effectively and easily treated by curettage and electrodesiccation. Small lesions (5–20 mm) of the nodular or cystic type may be treated satisfactorily by this method in most locations. Central facial BCCs and those of infiltrating, micronodular or morphealike histologic type are prone to recurrence if treated with curettage and desiccation. These lesions are, thus, better treated by methods, such as excision or Mohs microsurgery, that permit examination of the margins.[26] Cure rates have been reported as 97% to 98% with curettage and electrodesiccation for BCC.[27,28] Paradoxically, despite these high cure rates, histologic examination after curettage and electrodessication shows that some residual tumor is present in almost 30% of cases. Thus, cure must also depend on other factors, such as residual tumor cell mass, inflammatory reaction, and healing responses.[19]

Curettage and electrodessication can be used for small SCCs in situ and well-differentiated primary SCCs less than 1 cm in diameter. For larger and higher-risk tumors, microscopically controlled surgery is recommended.[28] These high-risk SCCs include lesions arising on scars; ears; lips; areas of radiation or thermal injury; chronic ulcers or sinuses; BD; non–sun-exposed sites; and large (>2 cm), thick (>4 mm), poorly differentiated and recurrent SCCs or those arising in immune-compromised patients.[19]

Because the procedure does not divide the upper dermis connective tissue network, healing is usually predictable and occurs in most cases with mild scarring. However, hypopigmentation or hypertrophic scar formation may occur, the latter particularly when the upper trunk is treated.[18]

PHOTODYNAMIC THERAPY

Photodynamic therapy (PDT) may be briefly defined as the use of cytotoxic oxygen radicals (primarily singlet oxygen) generated from photoactivated molecular species to achieve a therapeutic response. The necessary components are photoactivating light, an exogenous photosensitizer, tissue oxygen, and a target cell. Photosensitizers may be administered systemically as intact macrocycles or topically as prophotosensitizers, which are metabolized to photoactive macrocycles. A time period is required after drug administration to allow photosensitizer production and partitioning into targeted tissue and cellular compartments. Visible light from coherent (laser) or noncoherent sources is used to illuminate the skin. The light can be either low power, nonthermal, and continuous wave or high power, photothermal, and pulsed; the latter type introduces varying degrees of photothermal injury via biologic chromophores, augmenting overall clinical injury. Target cells may undergo apoptosis caused by membrane-bound photosensitizers or ischemic necrosis caused by vascular injury from photosensitizers concentrated in endothelial cells or both.[29] There is also evidence that PDT may act as a biologic response modifier.[30] PDT is a broadly inflammatory event; cytokines, chemokines, and other immunogenic proteins

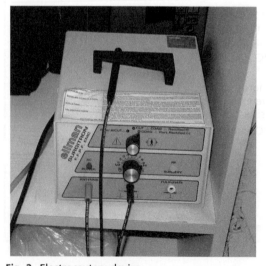

Fig. 2. Electrocautery device.

released by injured and dying cells create an inflammatory and immunologically active milieu.[29]

The most common and perhaps most sought-after oncologic indication for PDT remains BCC. Studies comparing its efficacy against standard therapies, such as cryosurgery, surgical excision, or Mohs micrographic surgery, are limited or absent. Systemic porphyrin-based PDT clearly showed that BCCs respond 80% to 100%, but these studies relied on short-term follow-up and clinical responses.[31,32] The systemic photosensitizer agents used to treat BCCs in the studies included porfimer sodium, benzoporphyrin derivative monoacid ring A, and meta-tetrahydroxyphenylchlorin, whereas 5-aminolevulinic acid (ALA) and methyl-esterified ALA (mALA) were the primary topical agents. Although response rates were encouraging with systemic PDT, there were several expected drawbacks, including generalized photosensitivity, facial edema, and pain. Topical approaches to the photodynamic treatment of BCC have been based almost entirely on ALA and more recently mALA. Topical photosensitization for PDT offers clinical advantages of ease of drug delivery and photosensitivity confined to the application site. No generalized photosensitivity occurs because of the limited systemic absorption of ALA or protoporphyrin IX. An attractive feature of topical PDT is the ability to treat relatively large body surface areas with a single intervention, often with a minimal amount of scarring.[29] Topical delivery of mALA proved effective in treating non-melanoma skin cancer. Three to six months after the PDT session, 87.5% (310 out of 350) of the BCCs responded completely. Ninety-three percent of BCCs received a single treatment session, 6% a second session.[33]

SCC in situ is also quite responsive to PDT. High cure rates have been observed with both systemic and topical photosensitizers. Few reports detail the photodynamic treatment of invasive cutaneous SCC and, thus far, the results have been unsatisfactory compared with surgical excision. Primary treatment of SCC with PDT should be reserved for early invasive disease (<1 mm) and must take advantage of multiple treatments and high doses of deeply penetrating red light. In advanced head and neck SCC, PDT should be considered an adjunctive treatment modality.[29,34] Reports of higher recurrence rates in NMSC suggest that photodynamic therapy may be best reserved for select situations when better-established methods are not feasible.[35]

RADIOTHERAPY

Radiotherapy (RT) consists of the use of ionizing radiation in the treatment of cancer via 2 main modalities: external RT and interstitial curietherapy. External RT uses low-energy X photons (contact x-ray therapy), high-energy X photons, gamma rays, or electron beams. It is a noninvasive form of treatment that may be used in SCC regardless of size or depth. Several sessions (mean: 10–30) are required over a period of 3 to 6 weeks. Dose fractionation achieves better cosmetic results while increasing treatment time. A safety margin of 1.0 to 1.5 cm around the tumor is recommended because of the risk of microscopic dissemination. RT exposes patients to the risk of a second carcinoma in the irradiated area. Interstitial curietherapy consists of implanting plastic tubes through which iridium 192 wires may be loaded into the tumor. During treatment, patients are hospitalized for 3 to 4 days in a specialized unit.[14] RT has been used in all forms of SCC and has displayed efficacy comparable with that of surgery, but because the most SCCs consist of small lesions, surgery has the advantage of ease of use, rapid wound healing, and with cosmetic results. The National Health and Medical Research Council's (NHMRC) guidelines, thus, recommend RT solely as a second-line treatment and in the following cases only[36]:

- A minority of primary SCC, when the patients' condition contraindicates surgery, the patients refuse surgery
- Recurring or advanced SCC when RT may be combined with surgery to improve tumor control
- Residual tumors where surgical treatment is unfeasible
- Management of metastases

According to the National Comprehensive Cancer Network's (NCCN) guidelines, RT may be indicated as a first-line treatment in patients older than 60 years for small primary SCC at sites other than hands, feet, or genital organs. RT may be considered an adjuvant to Mohs surgery in the event of extensive perineural invasion and is indicated in addition to incomplete excision of low-risk SCC. It is not recommended in verrucous SCC.[37]

RT can be used for the treatment of small BCCs or larger lesions when surgery will leave a poor functional or cosmetic result. It also has a role to play after primary surgery if the margins are ambiguous and further surgery is thought not to be appropriate for the patient. It should not be used for re-treating BCCs that have recurred after previous RT. The morpheic BCC subtype or the presence of underlying bone or cartilage involvement are relative contraindications for the use of radiation treatment. The technique and dose are the same for both BCC and SCC, but a wider margin is taken around the tumor in SCC and patients are subjected to a more frequent and longer follow-up as suggested in the British Association of Dermatology's guidelines.[38]

LASERS

Lasers induce coagulative necrosis, ablation, and hyperthermia leading to tumor destruction.[4] This therapy is rarely used to treat NMSC. Little evidence of its efficacy exists, and there are no comparisons with other treatment modalities.[18]

A few studies have provided evidence that lasers represent a new, effective treatment option for the management of NMSCs.[39–41]

Carbon dioxide (CO_2) lasers have been used to treat superficial BCCs and BD. The use of super-pulsed CO_2 lasers was studied in 44 patients with BD. The total response rate was 97.7%, and clearance after one treatment was achieved in 86.3% patients.[42] Moskalik and colleagues[41] performed a study on neodymium (Nd) lasers for the treatment of facial skin cancers. In 3461 patients with 3534 BCCs and 90 SCCs, pulsed Nd and Nd:YAG lasers were used and the patients were followed for 5 years. Recurrences were seen in 1.8% of patients with BCCs treated with a pulsed Nd laser, in 2.5% of patients with BCCs treated with an Nd:YAG laser, and in 4.4% of patients with SCCs treated with a pulsed Nd laser. They concluded that Nd lasers represent a useful way to treat facial skin cancers.

Laser is a costly and relatively inaccessible method. The data in the literature are insufficient to draw firm conclusion on its efficacy.[14]

TOPICAL 5-FU

It has been used for the treatment of AKs, superficial BCCs, and selected SCCs in situ.[35] It decreases cell proliferation and induces cellular death, particularly in cells with high mitotic rates, through inhibition of thymidylate synthetase, which interferes with DNA synthesis. Because of the lack of penetration through the dermis, 5-FU is generally not recommended for invasive BCCs and SCCs.[4] Several studies have reported the efficacy of topical 5-FU 5% ointment for the treatment of NMSC, with good to excellent cosmetic results; however, high recurrence rates have been frequently reported.[43,44] Oral 5-FU can be used also multiple or recurrent SCCs that had failed prior standard treatments.[45]

IMIQUIMOD

Imiquimod stimulates the innate and cell-mediated immune responses, potentiating antiviral, antitumoral, and immunoregulatory properties.[4] It activates cells of the innate immune system to secrete cytokines and assume an activated state by changing the expression of surface molecules involved in cell-cell interactions. Monocytes, macrophages, B cells, and dendritic cells are antigen-presenting cells that are targeted by imiquimod. One mechanism by which imiquimod may activate these target cells is by the activation of Toll-like receptors (TLRs), which are a family of pathogen recognition receptors located on the cell surface of innate immune cells, such as dendritic cells. Imiquimod has been reported to activate TLR 7.[1] The Food and Drug Administration approved imiquimod 5% cream for the treatment of warts, AKs, and superficial BCC mostly in patients in whom surgery is not an option.[4] As a noninvasive treatment modality, imiquimod may have some advantages over surgical procedures, especially in regard to cosmetic outcomes.[46] In the treatment of superficial BCCs, various treatment regimens were applied in the studies (twice daily, once daily, 5 times per week, 3 times per week), achieving responses up to 100%. Regimens with more frequent applications (once daily and twice daily) were associated with the best responses.[47,48] The responses with imiquimod cream in nodular BCC are not as high as those seen in superficial BCC. This type of treatment modality applies better for those patients in which surgery, RT, or cryotherapy is not an option. An evidence-based systematic review supports the use of topical imiquimod as a monotherapy for superficial BCC and SCC in situ.[4] Resiquimod is a TLR 7/8 agonist that has similar effects as imiquimod on monocytic cells, although it is 10 to 100 times more potent than imiquimod.[49]

RETINOIDS

Derivatives of vitamin A, retinoids are evolving as potential tools in the prevention of new BCCs and SCCs. Isotretinoin is considered the most effective retinoid for the prevention of nonmelanoma skin cancer.[2,50] Topical tretinoin has been shown to decrease the number of solar keratoses and may help prevent their progression to carcinoma. The retinoids' mechanism of action involves the tumor-promotion phase of carcinogenesis by inducing apoptosis, impeding proliferation, and stimulating differentiation or a combination of these processes.[2] Tazarotene, a receptor-selective retinoid for retinoic acid receptors, has shown some positive responses after daily application to BCCs for several months.[51]

CYTOKINES

Cytokines play a pivotal role in the immune system by modulating the development and function of humoral or cell-mediated responses to self or foreign antigens. Intralesional injection of IFN has shown some positive effects in the treatment of NMSCs. Alpha 2a and 2b are especially strong inhibitors of malignant cell growth and have demonstrated effectiveness, both individually and as combined agents, in the treatment of BCCs.[52] Several investigators have followed the injection protocol of 1.5 × 10^6 IU IFNα-2b three times a week (TIW) for 3 weeks (total dose of 13.5 × 10^6 IU).[13] In the sole placebo-controlled study, a cure rate of 81% at the 1-year follow-up was obtained. According to the results of this study, clinical signs of improvement in most tumors appear at 8 weeks and are marked at 16 weeks.[53] IFN may be also used to debulk large tumors.[54] Another use of IFNα-2b may be for the treatment of positive margins after surgical excision.[13]

CYCLOOXYGENASE-2 INHIBITORS

Increasing evidence is pointing to the role of cyclooxygenase-2 (COX-2) and its products, notably prostaglandin E2, in the development of NMSC. A specific COX-2 inhibitor, celecoxib, has shown potential therapeutic benefit in the prevention of cutaneous neoplasia. Oral and topical celecoxib have demonstrated a chemopreventive effect in animal studies by inhibiting new tumor formation and delaying tumor latency. Double-blinded, randomized, placebo-controlled trials in humans are warranted to define the role of COX-2 inhibitors in the prevention and treatment of NMSC.[2]

BETULINIC ACID

Betulin, betulinic acid, oleanolic acid, lupeol, and erythrodiol are pentacyclic triterpenes that have antiviral, antimicrobial, hepatoprotective, and anti-tumoral effects.[55,56] They promote keratinocyte differentiation and the induction of cytotoxic, anti-proliferative, and apoptotic effects on tumor cells.[57]

CYCLOPAMINE

It is a steroidal alkaloid extracted from the corn lily, *Veratrum californicum*, which is very common in subalpine meadows. It has shown inhibitory activity against the hedgehog family of intercellular signaling proteins. Because this membrane complex, particularly the Sonic Hedgehog subtype, has recently been implicated in the development of BCC, it may be an alternative treatment choice for NMSC. Clinical studies are needed to evaluate the efficacy and safety of topical cyclopamine for the treatment of NMSC.[4]

GDC-0449 (VISMODEGIB)

It is another hedgehog pathway inhibitor specifically targeting the proto-oncogene smoothened membrane protein. It is more potent and has favorable properties than cyclopamine.[4,58] Von Hoff and colleagues[59] reported that GDC-0449 had antitumor activity in patients with advanced BCC. Further clinical studies are needed to evaluate the safety and efficacy of GDC-0449 for the treatment of NMSC.

EPIDERMAL GROWTH FACTOR RECEPTOR INHIBITORS

The epidermal growth factor receptor gene codes for a transmembrane tyrosine kinase receptor related to cellular proliferation and epithelial development. Its overexpression has been associated with non–small cell lung cancer, colorectal cancer, and SCC.[4,14] Several antitumoral agents that block this receptor have been developed for the treatment of these cancers, including gefitinib and erlotinib. In addition, monoclonal antibodies, cetuximab and panitumumab, have been developed.[4] In a noncontrolled phase II study involving 103 patients with metastatic or recurring SCC of the head and neck, treated with cetuximab alone, the response rate was 13%.[60] It needs further controlled studies to assess the value of this drug.

AFAMELANOTIDE (CUV1647)

Ultraviolet B (UVB) induces the synthesis of melanin in melanocytes. The increase in melanin may have protective effects against UVB. Afamelanotide is an analogue of melanocyte stimulating hormone with higher potency and longer action than the naturally occurring hormone. It is currently being studied to evaluate its efficacy in reducing the number of AKs and SCCs.[4]

CAPECITABINE

It is an oral prodrug of 5-FU that has demonstrated efficacy for the treatment of SCC, particularly in combination with IFN. As a monotherapy, it was administered orally at a dose of 1 g/m^2 divided into 2 daily doses on days 1 through 14 of a 21-day treatment cycle in 14 transplant patients with recurrent SCCs and BCCs. It significantly decreased the recurrence rates in these patients.[4,61]

SUMMARY

The knowledge on nonsurgical therapies is still being raised for the treatment of NMSC. These patients should be evaluated individually according to the type, severity, location of the lesion, patient age, preference, and other circumstances. Although surgery is the gold standard for NMSC, nonsurgical management is effective and sometimes a preferable strategy for selected cases. New nonsurgical agents, such as imiquimod, reduced the morbidity and mortality of these patients.

Patients with skin cancer should be examined and receive multidisciplinary treatment. Nonsurgical treatment modalities should be kept in mind in appropriate cases. With further studies, new targeted agents will be developed for the management of NMSCs.

REFERENCES

1. Gaspari AA, Sauder DN. Immunotherapy of basal cell carcinoma: evolving approaches. Dermatol Surg 2003;29(10):1027–34.
2. Chakrabarty A, Geisse JK. Medical therapies for nonmelanoma skin cancer. Clin Dermatol 2004;22: 183–8.
3. Nyugen TH, Ho DQ. Nonmelanoma skin cancer. Curr Treat Options Oncol 2002;3:193–203.
4. Amini S, Viera MH, Valins W, et al. Nonsurgical innovations in the treatment of nonmelanoma skin cancer. J Clin Aesthet Dermatol 2010;3:20–34.
5. McGuire JF, Ge NN, Dyson S. Nonmelanoma skin cancer of the head and neck I: histopathology and clinical behavior. Am J Otolaryngol 2009;30(2): 121–33.
6. Seidler AM, Bramlette TB, Washington CV, et al. Mohs versus traditional surgical excision for facial and auricular nonmelanoma skin cancer: an analysis of cost-effectiveness. Dermatol Surg 2009;35(11): 1776–87.
7. Bagheri M, Safai B. Cutaneous malignancies of keratinocytic origin. Clin Dermatol 2001;19:244–52.
8. King SC, Chen S. Analyzing the cost of preventing nonmelanoma skin cancer. J Invest Dermatol 2009; 129(12):2745–6.
9. Gibbs P, Gonzalez R, Lee L, et al. Medical management of cutaneous malignancies. Clin Dermatol 2001;19:298–304.
10. Ho T, Byrne PJ. Evaluation and initial management of the patient with facial skin cancer. Facial Plast Surg Clin North Am 2009;17(3):301–7.
11. Ge NN, McGuire JF, Dyson S, et al. Nonmelanoma skin cancer of the head and neck II: surgical treatment and reconstruction. Am J Otolaryngol 2009; 30(3):181–92.
12. Lien MH, Sondak VK. Nonsurgical treatment options for basal cell carcinoma. J Skin Cancer 2011;2011: 571734 [Epub 2011 Jan 9].
13. Kim KH, Yavel RM, Gross VL, et al. Intralesional interferon α-2b in the treatment of basal cell carcinoma and squamous cell carcinoma: revisited. Dermatol Surg 2004;30:116–20.
14. Bonerandi JJ, Beauvillain C, Caquant L, et al. Guidelines for the diagnosis and treatment of cutaneous squamous cell carcinoma and precursor lesions. J Eur Acad Dermatol Venereol 2011;25(Suppl 5): 1–51.
15. Galiczynski EM, Vidimos AT. Nonsurgical treatment of nonmelanoma skin cancer. Dermatol Clin 2011; 29:297–309.
16. Robinson JK. Advances in the treatment of nonmelanoma skin cancer. Dermatol Clin 1991;9(4):757–64.
17. Rompel R. Dermatological surgery. In: Burgdorf WH, Plewig G, Landthaler M, editors. Braun-Falco's dermatology. 3rd edition. Italy: Springer Medizin Verlag Heidelberg; 2009. p. 1613–42.
18. Quinn AG, Perkins W. Non-melanoma skin cancer and other epidermal skin tumours. In: Burns T, Breathnach S, Cox N, et al, editors. Rook's textbook of dermatology, vol. 52, 8th edition. Oxford (United Kingdom): Blackwell Science; 2010. p. 1–48.
19. Lawrence CM, Telfer NR. Dermatological surgery. In: Burns T, Breathnach S, Cox N, et al, editors. Rook's textbook of dermatology, vol. 77, 8th edition. Oxford (United Kingdom): Blackwell Science; 2010. p. 1–50.
20. Kuflik EG, Gage AA. The 5 year cure rate achieved by cryosurgery for skin cancer. J Am Acad Dermatol 1991;24:1002–4.
21. Holt PJ. Cryotherapy for skin cancer: results over a 5 year period using liquid nitrogen spray cryosurgery. Br J Dermatol 1998;119:231–40.
22. Nordic P. Curettage-cryosurgery for nonmelanoma skin cancer of the external ear: excellent 5-year results. Br J Dermatol 1999;140:291–3.
23. Kuflik EG. Cryosurgery. In: Bolognia JL, Jorizzo JL, Papini RP, editors. Dermatology. 2nd edition. St. Louis: Elsevier Ltd; 2008. p. 2121–6.
24. Zacarian SA. Cryosurgery of cutaneous carcinomas: an 18-year study of 3022 patients with 4228 carcinomas. J Am Acad Dermatol 1983;9:947–56.
25. Odom RB, James WD, Berger TG. Dermatologic surgery. In: Andrews' diseases of the skin. 9th edition. Philadelphia: WB Saunders Co; 2000. p. 1073–90.
26. Odom RB, James WD, Berger TG. Epidermal nevi, neoplasms, and cysts. In: Andrews' diseases of the skin. 9th edition. Philadelphia: WB Saunders Co; 2000. p. 800–68.
27. Spiller WF, Spiller RF. Treatment of basal cell epithelioma by curettage and electrodessication. J Am Acad Dermatol 1984;11:808–14.

28. Ponten F, Lundeberg J, Asplund A. Principles of tumor biology and pathogenesis of BCCs and SCCs. In: Bolognia JL, Jorizzo JL, Papini RP, editors. Dermatology. 2nd edition. St. Louis: Elsevier Ltd; 2008. p. 1627–59.

29. Tope WD, Bhardwaj SS. Photodynamic therapy. In: Bolognia JL, Jorizzo JL, Papini RP, editors. Dermatology. 2nd edition. St. Louis: Elsevier Ltd; 2008. p. 2071–87.

30. Oseroff A. PDT as a cytotoxic agent and biological response modifier: implications for cancer prevention and treatment in immunosuppressed and immunocompetent patients. J Invest Dermatol 2006;126: 542–4.

31. Fritsch C, Goerz G, Ruzicka T. Photodynamic therapy in dermatology. Arch Dermatol 1998;134: 207–14.

32. Kalka K, Merk H, Mukhtar H. Photodynamic therapy in dermatology. J Am Acad Dermatol 2000;42: 389–413.

33. Soler AM, Warloe T, Berner A, et al. A follow up study of recurrence and cosmesis in completely responding superficial and nodular basal cell carcinomas treated with methyl 5-aminolevulinate-based photodynamic therapy alone and with prior curettage. Br J Dermatol 2001;145:467–71.

34. Dilkes MG, DeJode ML, Rowntree-Taylor A, et al. m-THPC photodynamic therapy for head and neck cancer. Lasers Med Sci 1996;11:23–9.

35. Rigel DS, Cockerell CJ, Carucci J, et al. Actinic keratosis, basal cell carcinoma and squamous cell carcinoma. In: Bolognia JL, Jorizzo JL, Papini RP, editors. Dermatology. 2nd edition. St. Louis: Elsevier Ltd; 2008. p. 1641–59.

36. Non melanoma skin cancer: guidelines for treatment and management in Australia. Clinical practice guidelines. Canberra (Australia): National Health Medical Research Council; 2002.

37. Clinical practice guidelines in oncology. Basal cell and squamous cell skin cancers. National Comprehensive Cancer Network. Available at: http://www. nccn.org/professionals/physician_gls/f_guidelines. asp. Accessed October 12, 2011.

38. Kelly CG, Peat I. Radiotherapy and reactions to ionizing radiation. In: Burns T, Breathnach S, Cox N, et al, editors. Rook's textbook of dermatology, vol. 79, 8th edition. Oxford (United Kingdom): Blackwell Science; 2010. p. 1–19.

39. Hantash BM, Stewart DB, Cooper ZA, et al. Facial resurfacing for non-melanoma skin cancer prophylaxis. Arch Dermatol 2006;142:976–82.

40. Iyer S, Friedli A, Bowes L, et al. Full face laser resurfacing: therapy and prophylaxis for actinic keratoses and nonmelanoma skin cancer. Lasers Surg Med 2004;34:114–9.

41. Moskalik K, Kozlov A, Demin E, et al. The efficacy of facial skin cancer treatment with high-energy pulsed neodymium and Nd: YAG lasers. Photomed Laser Surg 2009;27:345–9.

42. Covadonga Martinez-Gonzalez M, del Pozo J, Paradela S, et al. Bowen's disease treated by carbon dioxide laser. A series of 44 patients. J Dermatolog Treat 2008;19:293–9.

43. Epstein E. Fluorouracil paste treatment of thin basal cell carcinomas. Arch Dermatol 1985;121:207–13.

44. Bargman H, Hochman J. Topical treatment of Bowen's disease with 5-fluorouracil. J Cutan Med Surg 2003;7:101–5.

45. Cartei G, Cartei F, Interlandi G, et al. Oral 5-fluorouracil in squamous cell carcinoma of the skin in the aged. Am J Clin Oncol 2000;23:181–4.

46. Geisse J, Caro I, Lindholm J, et al. Imiquimod 5% cream for the treatment of superficial basal cell carcinoma: results from two phase III, randomized, vehicle-controlled studies. J Am Acad Dermatol 2004;50:722–33.

47. Beutner KR, Geisse JK, Helman D, et al. Therapeutic response of basal cell carcinoma to the immune response modifier imiquimod 5% cream. J Am Acad Dermatol 1999;41:1002–7.

48. Geisse JK, Rich P, Pandya A, et al. Imiquimod 5% cream for the treatment of superficial basal cell carcinoma: a double-blind, randomized, vehicle-controlled study. J Am Acad Dermatol 2002;47: 390–8.

49. Jones T. Resiquimod 3M. Curr Opin Investig Drugs 2003;4:214–8.

50. Niles RM. The use of retinoids in the prevention and treatment of skin cancer. Expert Opin Pharmacother 2002;3:299–303.

51. Peris K, Fargnoli MC, Chimenti S. Preliminary observations on the use of topical tazarotene to treat basal cell carcinoma. N Engl J Med 1999;341:1767–8.

52. Alpsoy E, Yilmaz E, Basaran E, et al. Comparison of the effects of intralesional interferon alfa-2a, 2b and the combination of 2a and 2b in the treatment of basal cell carcinoma. J Dermatol 1996;23:394–6.

53. Cornell RC, Greeenway HT, Tucker SB, et al. Intralesional interferon therapy for basal cell carcinoma. J Am Acad Dermatol 1990;23:694–700.

54. Stenquist B, Wennberg AM, Gisslen H, et al. Treatment of aggressive basal cell carcinoma with intralesional interferon: evaluation of efficacy by Mohs surgery. J Am Acad Dermatol 1992;27:65–9.

55. Jager S, Laszczyk MN, Scheffler A. A preliminary pharmacokinetic study of betulin, the main pentacyclic triterpene from extract of outer bark of birch (Betulae alba cortex). Molecules 2008;13:3224–35.

56. Krasutsky PA. Birch bark research and development. Nat Prod Rep 2006;23:919–42.

57. Huyke C, Reuter J, Rödig M, et al. Treatment of actinic keratoses with a novel betulin-based oleogel. A prospective, randomized, comparative pilot study. J Dtsch Dermatol Ges 2009;7:128–33.

58. Rudin CM. Beyond the scalpel: targeting hedgehog in skin cancer prevention. Cancer Prev Res (Phila) 2010;3:1–3.

59. Von Hoff DD, LoRusso PM, Rudin CM, et al. Inhibition of the hedgehog pathway in advanced-basal cell carcinoma. N Engl J Med 2009;361: 1164–72.

60. Bauman JE, Eaton KD, Martins RG. Treatment of recurrent squamous cell carcinoma of the skin with cetuximab. Arch Dermatol 2007;143:889–92.

61. Jirakulaporn T, Mathew J, Lindgren BR, et al. Efficacy of capecitabine in secondary prevention of skin cancer in solid-organ transplanted recipients (OTR). J Clin Oncol 2009;27:1519.

Nonmelanoma Skin Cancer of the Head and Neck
Surgical Treatment

Timur M. Akcam, MD[a,*], Wolfgang Gubisch, MD[b],
Halis Unlu, MD[c]

KEYWORDS

- Cutaneous cancer • Squamous cell carcinoma • Basal cell carcinoma • Nonmelonoma surgery
- Surgical excision • Skin cancer margin • Mohs micrographic surgery

KEY POINTS

- Define the risk factors of the tumor.
- Identify clinical margins under optimal lighting and magnification.
- Dermoscopy may be helpful to identify clinical margins better.
- In selected cases, prior curettage may help to delineate clinical margins; however, it is controversial.
- Mark surgical margins using scale before local anesthetic infiltration.
- For surgical excision, minimal surgical margin is recommended to be 3 to 4 mm for BBCs with well-defined clinical borders. Leave at least 4 to 6 mm healthy tissue around the SCCs.
- For the excision of high-risk tumors, prefer Mohs' micrographic surgery, if it is available.
- Surgical excision with intraoperative margin assessment with frozen section or preferably staged surgery can also be used safely.
- Do not perform complicated reconstructions without achieving tumor-free margins.
- In the management of incomplete excised NMSCs consider surgery primarily, and consider wait-and-see approach in selected cases.
- Late recurrences may occur; follow patients at least 5 years.

INTRODUCTION

The term "nonmelanoma skin cancer" (NMSC) is used to define basal cell carcinoma (BCC) and squamous cell carcinoma (SCC) of the skin, and other rare primary cutaneous malignancies. Because most NMSCs originate from the epidermis, the upper layer of the skin, it is often detected at an early stage and can be treated locally. Treatment of NMSC can be broadly classified into surgical and nonsurgical treatment. Surgical excision is the most effective treatment option for most NMSCs. This article focuses on surgical treatment for NMSC; repair of the defect after excision is beyond the scope of this article.

The treatment of a facial skin cancer aims to achieve complete eradication of the cancer with a good and acceptable cosmetic and functional outcome; however, complete eradication of the tumor should be the primary goal. Although

The Authors of this article declare that they have no professional or financial affiliations for themselves or their spouse/partner to disclose.

[a] Department of Otorhinolaryngology, Head and Neck Surgery, Gulhane Military Medical Academy, General Tevfik Saglam Caddesi, Etlik Kecioren, Ankara 06018, Turkey; [b] Department of Plastic and Reconstructive Surgery, Marien Hospital, Böheimstasse 37, Stutgard 70199, Germany; [c] Department of Otorhinolaryngology, Head and Neck Surgery, Ekol Hospital, 8019/16 Sokak No:4 Cigli-Izmir, Turkey
* Corresponding author.
E-mail addresses: takcam@gata.edu.tr; takcam@gmail.com

facialplastic.theclinics.com

surgery is the treatment of choice for high-risk NMSCs, low-risk NMSCs may be treated by either nonsurgical or surgical treatment options. Therefore, the most important step in the treatment planning of the NMSCs is to determine if the tumor has high risk or low risk to recur or metastasize. Presence of characteristics associated with recurrence or metastasis make a tumor high risk, whereas a tumor that is unlikely to recur or metastasize is determined to be low risk.

RISK FACTORS OF RECURRENCE AND METASTASES

- Location
- Size
- Histologic subtype
- Degree of differentiation
- Tumor thickness/Depth of invasion
- Perineural and Lymphovascular invasion
- Immunosuppression
- Recurrence

Location

Location of the tumor is one of the most important factors affecting the outcome of treatment of NMSCs. Certain sites of the head and neck region are more likely to recur and metastasize.[1–6]

Swanson[6] illustrated high-risk locations of face as an "H" zone, because of the higher recurrence rate and the functional and cosmetic importance (**Fig. 1**). Recurrences are most commonly seen on nose, cheek, auricular area, periocular area, scalp, and forehead.[4,5] SCCs located on ear, temple, forehead, and anterior scalp that drain to parotid gland and lower lip are associated with higher incidence of metastases.[7]

Size

Lesion size is also an important prognostic risk factor for NMSCs and larger tumors have higher recurrence rates.[8–11] The degree of subclinical extension was unpredictable in tumors 2 cm or larger in diameter when compared with tumors less than 2 cm in diameter.[12] The horizontal diameter of BCCs is an important factor for tumor invasion; a tumor with larger diameters invades more deeply.[8] The lesion size of SCC was found to be associated with recurrence and depth of invasion.[10] Furthermore, lesion size 4 cm or greater was one of the most significant factors that diminished disease-specific survival. In another study, tumor size greater than 2 cm was found to be an independent risk factor for recurrence-free survival.[11] Cherpelis and colleagues[13] showed that tumor size significantly correlated with metastasis, with increasing risk for tumors larger than 2 cm in size, and they proposed

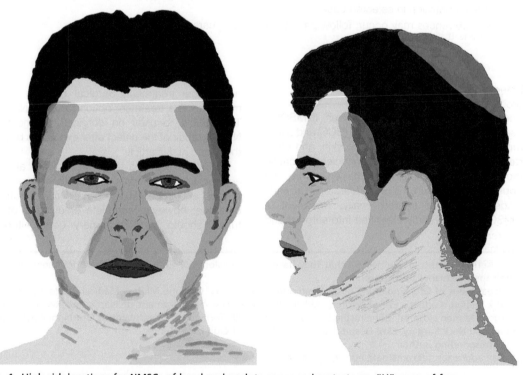

Fig. 1. High-risk locations for NMSCs of head and neck to recur and metastases, "H" zone of face.

that invasive SCCs that are smaller than 1 cm in size may metastasize, but it is uncommon.

Histologic Subtype

Histologic subtypes of NMSCs are a predictor of risk of recurrence and metastasis. The most potent predictor of recurrence for BCCs was found to be aggressive histologic type of the tumor, besides positive excision margins.[14] Any histologic variant of BCC may be locally aggressive and metastasize, but metatypical and basosquamous, morpheaform, infiltrating, and micronodular subtypes of BCC are more prone to exhibit an aggressive behavior.[15] Infiltrative, morpheic, and micronodular subtypes of BCC show locally aggressive behavior and invade more deeply than nodular BCCs.[8] On eyelid, 29.41% of patients with fibrous or sclerozing BCC, referred to as infiltrative, superficial multicentric, or morpheo growth pattern, recurred, whereas only 2.38% of nodular BCCs recurred.[16]

Clinical behaviors of subtypes of SCCs also vary widely, although all squamoid neoplasms are commonly referred as generic SCC. Desmoplastic growth pattern of SCC is an independent risk factor for local recurrence.[17] Cassarino and colleagues[18] made a clinicopathologic classification of cutaneous SCC according to metastatic rate in which tumors were separated as low risk (≤2% metastatic rate); intermediate risk (3%–10% metastatic rate); high risk (>10% metastatic rate); and intermediate behavior (insufficient data to determine the metastatic risk) (**Table 1**).

Degree of Differentiation

Differentiation of the tumor is also an important prognostic criterion for cutaneous SCC. Poorly

differentiated SCCs tend to present more locally aggressive behavior and demonstrate increased recurrence rates compared with well-differentiated SCCs.[11,19] There is also a higher propensity to develop regional metastases in poorly differentiated SCCs.[7]

Tumor Thickness and Depth of Invasion

Tumor thickness or depth of invasion is another important prognostic predictor of SCCs. Deep invasion diminishes disease-specific survival in cutaneous SCCs.[10] Brantsch and colleagues[17] found tumor thickness of SCC greater than 6 mm to be an independent risk factor for local recurrence and proposed to divide SCC into three main risk categories for metastasis according to tumor thickness: (1) no detectable risk (≤2 mm tumor thickness); (2) low risk (2–6 mm tumor thickness); and (3) high risk (>6 mm tumor thickness). Metastatic SCCs are more likely to be deeper (Clark level V).[13] Depth of invasion greater than 4 mm is associated with an increasing risk of metastases.[7]

Perineural and Lymphovascular Invasion

Perineural invasion diminishes disease-specific survival in cutaneous SCCs[10] and was found to be an independent risk factor for overall and recurrence-free survival of cutaneous SCC of the head and neck.[20] Presence of lymphovascular invasion may also increase the risk of developing nodal metastases.[7]

Immunosuppression

SCC of skin behaves more aggressive in patients who are immunosuppressed than in patients who are immunocompetent,[21–23] and has higher

Table 1
Clinicopathologic classification of cutaneous SCC according to metastatic rate

Low-Risk SCC Types I	Intermediate-Risk Types	High-Risk Tumors	Intermediate Category
SCC arising in actinic keratoses	Adenoid (acantholytic) SCC	Invasive Bowen disease	Clear cell SCC
Human papilloma virus–associated SCC,	Intraepidermal epithelioma with invasion	Adenosquamous carcinoma	Signet ring cell SCC
Tricholemmal carcinoma	Lymphoepithelioma-like carcinoma of the skin	Malignant proliferating pillar tumor	Papillary SCC
Spindle cell SCC		Desmoplastic SCC	Pigmented SCC
		De novo SCC	Follicular SCC
		SCC arising in association with predisposing factors	SCC arising from benign sweat gland cysts
			Squamoid eccrine ductal carcinoma

Data from Cassarino DS, Derienzo DP, Barr RJ. Cutaneous squamous cell carcinoma: a comprehensive clinicopathologic classification. Part one. J Cutan Pathol 2006;33:191–206.

metastatic potential.[21] Although the recurrence rate of SCC and BCC was found to be similar after renal transplantation, 48% and 42.8%, respectively,[21] any role of immunosuppression on aggressive behavior that has been shown for SCC has not been proved for BCC.[22,23]

Recurrent Tumor

Recurrent tumors have more extensive subclinical spread.[3] The incidence of incomplete excision of BCC was 3.7% in primary lesions, but it was 13.1% in the recurrent lesions.[24]

Site of Chronic Wound and Burn Scar

SCCs arising at the site of chronic wound or burn scar have three times diminished 5-year recurrence-free survival compared with SCCs as a whole (28% vs 74%).[11]

SURGICAL TREATMENT OPTIONS

There are three margin concepts to differentiate in the treatment of NMSCs: (1) clinical margin, (2) surgical margin, and (3) pathologic margin (**Fig. 2**). Clinical margin defines the visible borders of a tumor. However, the clinical margin of a tumor does not necessarily refer to histopathologic borders of the tumor, namely pathologic margin. Tumor may have some amount of subclinical extension that cannot be identified visibly. Therefore, excised specimen must incorporate sufficient amount of normal tissue around the tumor to prevent recurrences. The preferred excision margin of a tumor with some amount of normal-appearing tissue defines the surgical margin. However, one must also avoid removing excessive tissue to spare normal tissue in order not to disturb cosmesis and function. Therefore, determining surgical margins of a tumor is crucial in the surgical treatment of NMSC.

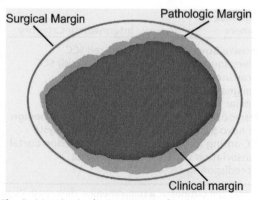

Fig. 2. Margins in the treatment of a skin cancer.

Identification of lesions with extensive subclinical spread preoperatively helps surgeon to determine the optimal surgical procedure and surgical margin. Batra and Kelley[3] performed a retrospective study to develop a scale to predict extensive subclinical spread of NMSCs. Analyses of 1095 BCCs and SCCs revealed that the significant predictors of extensive subclinical spread of NMSCs are basosquamous, morpheaform, nodular, and recurrent subtypes located on the nose; morpheaform BCC on the cheek; any tumor on the eyelid, temple, or ear helix; any tumor on the neck in men; recurrent BCC in men; and preoperative size less than 10 mm.[3]

The surgical procedures used in the treatment of NMSCs aim to remove the tumor with a tumor-free surrounding tissue. This may be achieved by either surgical excision with standard margins; surgical excision with frozen-section margin assessment; surgical excision with delayed repair (staged surgery); or Mohs micrographic surgery (MMS). The comparison of these options regarding advantages and disadvantages is summarized in **Table 2**.

Surgical Excision with Standard Margins

This traditional surgical treatment is based on the removal of tumor relying on the clinical margins. Therefore, this approach is preferred for the treatment of tumors with well-defined clinical margins. Surgical excision with standard margins is indicated mostly in the treatment of low-risk NMSCs.

In most cases, tumors can be excised under local anesthesia. Identifying the clinical margin of the tumor preoperatively is crucial. The lesion is carefully inspected under optimal lighting ideally with magnification and palpated to determine the exact clinical margin of the tumor. The clinical margin, the assessed outline of the tumor, is dotted with ink or fine-tipped marking pen, and then the surgical margin is marked according to preferred peripheral clearance margin. Preoperative margin detection by digital dermoscopy may obtain better results to achieve safe margins.[25–27] Curettage before excision of NMSC may also be used to delineate margins of the tumor. Curettage before excision decreased the surgical failure rate for BCC by 24%, but did not decreased the rate for SCC.[28] It is advised to use a measurement of scale for marking the surgical margins. If the lesions are marked using only the naked eye, there is a tendency to underestimate surgical margins for large lesions and to overestimate for small lesions.[29] It was shown that marking surgical margins with aid of magnification reduces the incidence of incomplete resection.[30] Marking the relaxed skin tension lines is beneficial to obtain

Table 2
Comparisons of surgical options regarding advantages and disadvantages

Surgical Excision with Standard Margin	Surgical Excision with Frozen Section	Surgical Excision with Delay Repair	Mohs Micrographic Surgery
Relies on clinical margins	Relies on vertical frozen section assessment	Relies on permanent section assessment	Relies on horizontal frozen section assessment
Subtotal margin control (changes depending on the type of sectioning)	Subtotal margin control (changes depending on the type of sectioning)	Subtotal margin control (changes depending on the type of sectioning)	100% microscopically controlled margin
No special training and facilities required	Requires pathologist intraoperatively	No special training and facilities required	Special training and facilities required
Results in larger defect size	Results in larger defect size	Results in larger defect size (smaller when narrow margin is used)	Results in smaller defect size
Shorter operation time	Time-consuming operation	Shorter operation time (only for the excision)	Time-consuming operation
Re-excision may be required	Re-excision may be required (less than surgical excision and surgical excision with delay repair)	Re-excision may be required	No re-excision after operation
Reconstruction at the time of excision	Reconstruction at the time of excision	Reconstruction at a second stage	Reconstruction at the time of excision (if another reconstructive surgeon is not required)
Complicated reconstructions cannot be performed safely	Complicated reconstructions can be performed more safely	Complicated reconstructions can be performed most safely	Complicated reconstructions can be performed most safely
Least expense	Less expense	Increased expense	Increased expense
Relatively worse outcome	Better outcome	Best outcome	Best outcome

the orientation of incision to hide within a normal wrinkle.

Local anesthetic agent infiltration must be performed after assessing the clinical margin of the tumor in order not to impair the assessment. The lesion is excised by adhering exactly to the edge of the drawn surgical margin. The tumor is excised down into the subcutaneous fat, or adjacent involved anatomic layer (**Fig. 3**). Surgical excision provides a single specimen to evaluate the involvement of peripheral and deep margins by the tumor. The excised specimen should be marked for orientation during histopathologic assessment of the surgical margins by either sutures or different colors of tissue dyes. Safety of margins is checked by the pathologist postoperatively with permanent sectioning.

Wolf and Zitelli[31] showed that a minimum margin of 4 mm was necessary to totally eradicate well-defined bordered, primary BCCs with a diameter less than 2 cm, in more than 95% of cases. Significant correlation is present between the size of the lesion and margin involvement; incomplete excision is seen almost three times more in tumors greater than 2 cm in diameter.[12]

Narrow-margin elliptical excision with surgical margins up to 3 mm was found to be only 80% effective in achieving tumor-free margins.[32] However, Bisson and colleagues[33] compared the surgical margins and histologic margins of BCCs and found that in cases where the tumor was larger than they had anticipated, the discrepancy was never greater than 3 mm. They concluded that 3 mm surgical margin was sufficient for the

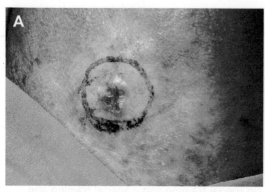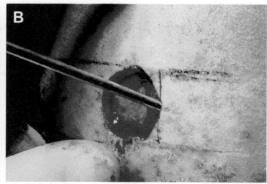

Fig. 3. BCC located on scalp. (*A*) Preferred surgical margin marked. (*B*) The lesion was excised down to the periosteum.

complete resection of the tumor. Griffiths and colleagues[34] propounded that 1- to 2-mm histologic margins may generally be considered adequate and to achieve such histologic clearance, clinical margins of 2 to 3 mm are required to allow tissue shrinkage. As the surgical margins are reduced, the incidence of incomplete excision increases.[24,35] Gulleth and colleagues[35] showed that increasing the size of margins decreased recurrence rates linearly until it reached 5 mm, which had the lowest recurrence rate. There was no significant change in the rate of tumor-free margins between 3- and 5-mm surgical margins, but recurrence rates decreased.

Minimal margins of excision around the clinical borders of SCC were recommended to be 4 mm margins in low-risk tumors, whereas at least a 6-mm margin for high-risk tumors was proposed.[36] Thomas and coworkers[37] showed that a surgical margin of 4 mm achieved an optimal excision beyond one microscopic high-power field in 96% of BCCs and in 97% of SCCs. They proposed to excise NMSCs less than 2 cm in diameter with a 4-mm margin of normal-appearing skin under magnification.

Unlu and colleagues[38] excised BCCs located on head and neck according to either "inspected healthy margins" visible on outer margins of the erythema or induration area surrounding the tumor or "safety margins," 2-mm margin for tumors less than 1 cm in size and 4-mm margin for tumors greater than 1 cm in size. Comparisons revealed that incomplete excision rates with inspected healthy margins and safety margins were similar for tumors less than 1 cm and greater than 1 cm in size. They recommended excising just what was seen, especially at the perioral, periorbital, and nasal regions where morbidity might be a problem.

Surgical excision with preferred margins is a good treatment option, especially for small NMSCs (**Fig. 4**). It shortens the operation time and costs less compared with other surgical options; however, multiple re-excisions may be needed, so the cost increases. Surgical margins should be determined according to pathologic characteristics, size, and location of the tumor. Surgical margin of 3 to 4 mm seems sufficient for most of the tumors. Safety margins of SCCs should be at least 4 to 6 mm. When the tumor is larger than 2 cm in diameter, has poorly defined borders, and high-risk to recur or metastases, it is better to prefer other treatment options. Otherwise, surgical margins should be increased. Because of the possibility of re-excisions, simple excision with permanent section margin assessment is usually preferred for lesions that can be repaired by primary closure.

Surgical Excision with Frozen Section Margin Assessment

Intraoperative frozen sectioning of NMSC is an effective tool to obtain tumor-free margins. If there is concern about the complete excision of the lesion, peripheral or deep biopsies are taken for intraoperative assessment of the histologic margins with frozen sections. The indications for frozen section examination in skin cancers are presence of poorly defined clinical margins, histopathologic types with infiltrative growth pattern, longstanding large or recurrent lesions, and tumors located in areas where skin preservation is desirable or arising near the planes of embryonic closure (**Fig. 5**).[39] Before extensive reconstructive surgeries, frozen sectioning is often used to ensure that margins are negative.

Surgical excision is performed standard fashion; however, proper orientation of the margins is crucial. To obtain an appropriate communication between the surgeon and pathologist, different color dyes or sutures are used to identify the margins of the tumor. There are three methods for sectioning of the skin specimen.[39] Representative perpendicular sectioning method does not fully survey the

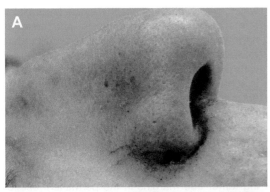

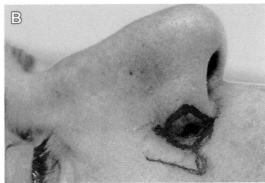

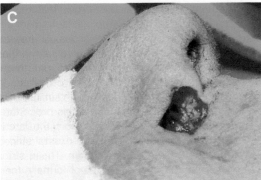

Fig. 4. (*A*) A small (<1 cm) BCC located on alar-facial junction. (*B*) Surgical margin marked. (*C*) Lesion excised completely.

peripheral margins, thus this method is inadequate. Traditional method of sectioning obtains vertical sections much like the slices of bread. Smaller specimens (<1–2 cm) are most appropriate for this technique. The variants of vertical section include breadloaf sectioning, cross-sectioning, breadloaf–cross-sectioning, and peripheral sectioning.[40]

Although breadloaf–cross-sectioning is superior to breadloaf sectioning and cross-sectioning, none of these methods fully survey margins (**Fig. 6**). The peripheral sectioning method evaluates lateral margins of a tumor, but not the deep margin. For larger specimens (>2 cm), en face method is best used.[39] Entire peripheral margins and deep margins

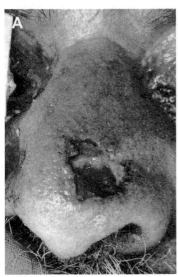

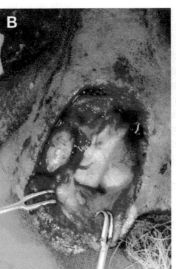

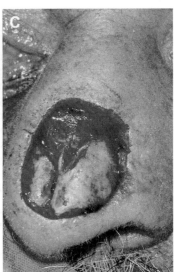

Fig. 5. (*A*) BCC located on the nose, high-risk area. (*B*) The lesion excised down to alar cartilages. (*C*) Not to excise too much tissue, frozen section margin assessment was used and cartilage structure is preserved.

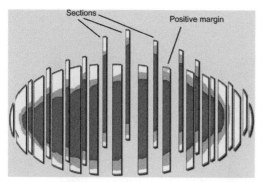

Fig. 6. Breadloaf sectioning. It is possible not to obtain sections from the positive margins with vertical horizontal sections.

are submitted en face for the evaluation of the margins. This technique provides a more accurate margin assessment, but the tumor's relationship to margin cannot be evaluated. If a positive margin is reported, re-excisions with frozen section margin assessment are performed until a tumor-free margin is obtained. It is recommended to submit the margins en face, if the additional tissue is less than 0.5 cm in width and greater than 1 cm in length. The tissue submitted should not be larger than 1 × 1 cm.[39]

The accuracy of frozen sections in detecting the presence or absence of tumor involvement at the surgical margins for skin cancers compared with permanent sections ranges between 72% and 91.1%.[41,42] False-negative results were obtained in 18.7% and 15.4% of BCCs and SCCs, respectively, in the primary excisions, whereas false-negative results were significantly lower in the residual tumors.[43] Kimyai-Asadi and colleagues[44] found that serial transverse cross-sectioning of the specimen with 4-mm intervals is only 44% sensitive for detecting residual tumor at the surgical margin when well-defined facial BCC is excised with 2-mm surgical margins. The larger the surgical margin being evaluated with frozen section, the greater the possibility of overlooked tumor cells and the incidence of recurrence. It is important to remember that negative surgical margins with frozen section assessment only represent the sampling of the margins.

Surgical Excision with Delayed Repair (Staged Surgery)

Simple excision with permanent margin assessment can also be performed with delayed repair.[45–48] If flaps or grafts are required for the reconstruction, to ensure that tumor-free margins are obtained, reconstruction can be delayed. Staged surgery may also be used for cases in which preservation of healthy tissue is crucial in terms of function and cosmesis, and therefore narrow margin excision is preferred.[46] Standard excision technique is used to excise the tumor with preferred surgical margin. After hemostasis is achieved, the wound is covered with nonadherent surgical dressing until permanent sectioning of the tumor is examined. If permanent sections of the specimen reveal tumor-free margins, reconstruction is performed; otherwise, subsequent excisions are performed until clearance of margins is obtained. It should be kept in mind that obtaining tumor-free margins in the permanent section assessment does not always prove that margin clearance is obtained. Pathologists traditionally examine only the margins of the slides of the specimen, not the entire margin. However, other than traditional histopathologic evaluation, three-dimensional histology may also be used to examine the entire margin when a skin tumor is excised with a certain margin. In this procedure, first a vertical strip is prepared from the lateral margin of the specimen; later a horizontal strip is cut from the base of the specimen. These strips are flattened and fixed in 60°C hot formalin for 2 hours. Then, they are embedded in paraffin and sectioned according to routine procedures. Twenty hours later, hematoxylin-eosin–stained slides are examined. The recurrence rates of three-dimensional histology-guided surgery seem similar to MMS.[49]

Excision of BCCs with 1- to 2-mm surgical margins required re-excision in 18% of the cases located on the face with delayed repair; a mean 5-year follow-up showed that 3% of the cases recurred in staged surgery.[45] In another study, with a wider margin (usually 3–5 mm) 8.2% of BCCs required a second-stage excision and 0.78% recurrence was reported in the average follow-up period of 20.37 months.[48]

Mohs Micrographic Surgery

The idea of removing neoplasms in a microscopically controlled serial manner with in situ fixation was conceived by Dr Frederic E. Mohs in the 1930s accidentally while studying the potential curative effects of substances into different neoplasms.[50] This fixed tissue technique was initially named "chemosurgery." However, after several improvements fresh tissue technique that eliminated most of the significant disadvantages of fixed tissue technique came into use, and finally the procedure was renamed MMS.[50]

The procedure of MMS, which allows the surgeon to examine peripheral margins 360 degrees around and deep margin, can be used in the surgical treatment of all NMSCs. Communication problems among surgeon and pathologist in the evaluation of margins are not an issue in MMS, because the Mohs surgeon also serves as the pathologist. It is typically the treatment of choice for high-risk BCCs and SCCs. NMSCs displaying any of the characteristics associated with higher recurrence or metastasis risk compose the indications of MMS (**Box 1**).

The procedure is typically well tolerated under local anesthesia; however, monitored sedation or general anesthesia can also be used in selected cases. Defining and marking the clinical margins of the tumor with a surgical pen under optimal lighting is the first step of the procedure. Marking significant anatomic and functional units may have benefits. Next, the area is anesthetized with local anesthetic infiltration. Curettage may also be used to debulk tumor, scraping away the poorly adherent tumor cells. However, the benefit of the curettage is controversial. Ratner and Bagiella[51] advocate that curettage decreases the number of Mohs surgical stages required for clearance of BCC, and thus decreases the operative time and increases the operative efficiency. Supporting this idea, Chung and colleagues[52] showed that the estimation of SCC and BCC tumor size and shape with curettage was 15 times more accurate than with usual and tactile assessment alone; nodular BBCs and SCCs were found to have greater potential to benefit from curettage than infiltrative BCCs. Contrary to these, Jih and colleagues[53] concluded that the curette had a limited role as a tumor-defining instrument and preoperative curettage did not reduce the number of stages of MMS required to attain histologic clearance of an NMSC. Furthermore, they propounded that although sparing of tissue is of significant concern, curettage may unnecessarily

---

Box 1
Indications for MMS

- Subtypes with infiltrative growth pattern
- Poorly defined clinical margins
- Located in high-risk anatomic sites of face
- Tumors greater than 2 cm in diameter
- Incompletely excised tumors
- Recurrent tumors
- Immunosuppressed patients
- Presence of perineural invasion, lymphovascular invasion
- Tumors arising at the site of chronic wound or scar

---

enlarge the surgical defect. The evidence that performing curettage before MMS results in a larger defect supports this opinion.[54]

After the final clinical borders are settled, incision of the first layer is performed with narrow surgical margins (usually 1–3 mm), using a scalpel positioned at a 45-degree angle to the skin. To orient the excised tissue accurately, markings extending onto the surrounding tissue are made by either scoring of tissue with scalpel or using gentian violet marker. Both methods can be used safely without resulting in scar tissue in scoring with scalpel or loss of orientation in gentian violet marker.[55] It is best to make markings at 12-o'clock and 6-o'clock positions for smaller excision, at additionally 3-o'clock and 9-o'clock positions for larger excisions (**Fig. 7A**), and at the acute angle of the specimen for piriform and fusiform excisions.[56] Incision is carried down to the level of subcutaneous fat and tumor is excised in the same plane in a horizontal fashion, parallel to the surface of the skin (**Fig. 7B**). MMS surgery is usually performed using a scalpel with #15 blade; however, flexible blade is alternatively offered to excise the deep margins.[57] Then, the specimen is sectioned to smaller pieces depending on tumor size. The skin edges are stained with different color dyes to indicate each edge and to preserve the orientation with the Mohs map, the schematic drawing of excision site.

Painted specimens are flattened so that superficial surface of the tissue is laid down in the same plane as the deeper surface (**Fig. 7C**). After the specimen is embedded and frozen in the medium, slices are prepared horizontally from the deeper surface of each sample of tissue (**Fig. 7D**). The number of slices and average thickness of each slice varies depending on the preferences of the surgeon; however, three and six slices with an average thickness of 5 to 6 μm are preferred.[56] Each section is evaluated correlating color dyes with the Mohs map so that the residual tumor can be localized, if present (**Fig. 7E**). In the event of residual tumor persistence, re-excisions are performed in the involved area and specimens are reviewed in the same way until all margins are clear (**Fig. 7F–H**). After clearance of the entire peripheral and deep margin is provided, the defect is reconstructed in the proper way. MMS ensures safety of margins quite effectively and reliably on the face (**Figs. 8** and **9**). Campbell and colleagues[58] evaluated the surgical margins with permanent histopathologic sections after "clear margins" were obtained by MMS and found that only 0.3% of cases contained persistent tumor.

The prospective, noncomparative studies revealed that the mean number of levels required

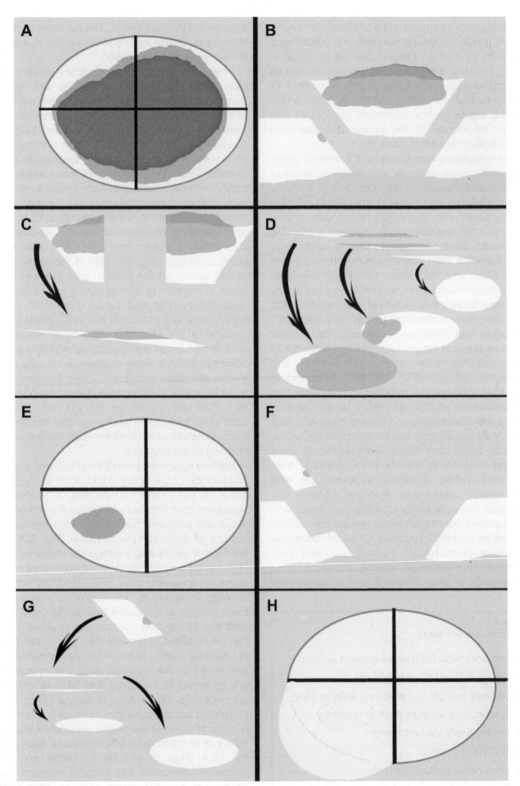

Fig. 7. Mohs micrographic surgery. (*A*) Tumor marked at the quarters. (*B*) Skin incised with 45-degree angle and excised through the level of subcutaneous fat. Specimen is sectioned to smaller pieces. (*C*) After skin edges are stained, specimen is flattened. (*D*) Slices are prepared horizontally from the deeper surface. Each section is evaluated in correlation with the Mohs map. (*E*) There is a residual tumor persistence in a quarter. (*F*) Re-excision is performed from the involved area. (*G*) Specimen of the second stage is examined in the same manner. (*H*) Margin clearance is achieved.

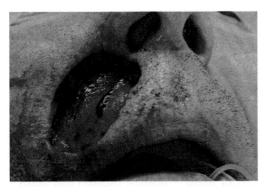

Fig. 8. BCC located on nasolabial fold excised with MMS.

for complete tumor eradication was 1.73 (median, 2) for BCC[59] and 1.60 (median, 1) for SCC.[4] Orengo and colleagues[60] achieved tumor-free margins in 74.3% of BCCs in the first two stages of MMS, when 1- to 2-mm narrow margins were used. Similar to this study, MMS with 2- to 3-mm margins eradicated tumor cells in 71% of BCCs within two Mohs stages.[61] BBCs that require more than two stages are mostly aggressive subtypes.[60] Recurrent tumors also require significantly more stages to achieve tumor-free margins.[4,59] MMS with 3-mm margins needed more than three stages to obtain histologic clearance in 22% of recurrent BCCs.[62] Increase in number of stages may be assumed to be disturbing for the patient; on the contrary, more intraoperative Mohs levels were found to be a predictor of higher short- and long-term satisfaction.[63] Probably, patients perceive themselves better cared for and treated as the number of stages increases.

Five-year recurrence rates of BBC after MMS for 5-year follow-up period ranges between 2.6% and 4.5%.[5,61,64] Recurrence rates of recurrent tumors are higher than primary tumors (1.4%–3.2% vs 4%–6.7%).[5,61,64] Smeets and colleagues[61] found that the 7-year recurrence rate of primary BCC

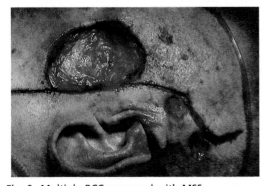

Fig. 9. Multiple BCCs removed with MSS.

was the same as the 5-year recurrence rate, but the 7-year recurrence rate of recurrent BCC (16%) was much higher than the 5-year recurrence rate (6.7%). Aggressive subtypes of BCC, large defect size (>4 cm in diameter), and four or more Mohs stages were found to be predictive for probability of recurrence.[61] Because a large proportion of recurrent BCCs recurred after 5 years of follow-up period, they recommended a follow-up period of 5 years for primary BCCs and 10 years for recurrent BCCs.[61]

Leibovitch and colleagues[4] designed a prospective, noncomparative, multidisciplinary study in which 1263 patients who underwent MMS for SCC were included. Most of these tumors (96.5%) were located on the head and neck. Of those, 381 cases were followed for 5 years and overall recurrence rate was found to be 3.9%, whereas it was 2.6% and 5.9% for primary and recurrent SCCs, respectively.[4]

Surgical Excision Versus MMS

Recurrence

Recurrence rate of NMSCs after treatment is an important issue that should be taken into consideration in treatment decision making. Five-year recurrence rate of NMSCs was found to be 4% for excision and 2.6% for MMS, using survival analysis.[65] In a prospective, randomized study 408 primary facial BCCs and 204 recurrent facial BCCs were assigned to the treatment of surgical excision or MMS. Of primary BCCs, seven after surgical excision and four after MMS recurred during the median follow-up period of 60 months; 5-year recurrence rates estimated by Kaplan-Meier analysis were 4.1% for surgical excision and 2.5% for MSS.[62] The percentages of recurrence of recurrent BBCs were 12.1% and 2.4% for surgical excision and MSS, respectively. The difference in the recurrence rates after surgical excision and MSS was significant for only recurrent facial BCCs. Although recurrence rate after surgical excision was higher than after MSS, the difference was not significant for primary facial BCCs.[62] In another prospective randomized controlled trial in which 397 primary facial BCCs and 204 recurrent BCCs were included, of primary BBCs, five (3%) after surgical excision and three (2%) after MMS recurred, whereas among the recurrent BBCs only three (3%) recurred after surgical excision.[66] Although MMS slightly lowered the recurrence rate for primary and recurrent tumors compared with surgical excision, the mean follow-up periods for primary and recurrent BCCs were only 2.66 years and 2.06 years, respectively, too short periods of time for all recurrences to occur. In another study, the recurrence rate of NMSCs after surgical excision and MMS was reported to be 0.98 and 0.75, respectively, which is much lower than other studies. However, the median follow-up periods were even shorter, 16 months and 24 months for surgical excision and MMS, respectively.[67] Recurrences can occur even after 5 years of follow-up.[62] Median time of detection of recurrence was 4.2 years, whereas recurrences were detected later after MMS than after surgical excision.[65] Therefore, it should be kept in mind that shorter follow-up periods do not represent the accurate recurrence rates of NMSCs or the success of a treatment option.

Tumor-free margins
The other important goal of surgical treatment is to achieve tumor-free margins using the most tissue-sparing method. Preservation of healthy tissue as much as possible lessens the need for complicated repair techniques, and so improves the cosmetic outcome besides saving time and cost. Therefore, providing smaller defect gains superiority of one surgical approach over the other. When standard 3-mm margins were used for MMS and surgical excision of BCC, overall defect sizes did not differ regarding surgical technique for primary and recurrent tumors after single excision and after single-stage of MMS.[66] In cases of incomplete excision, when re-excisions were performed or multiple MMS stages were required, comparison of defect sizes revealed significantly smaller defect sizes in favor of MMS.[66] NMSCs were controlled with 2- to 3-mm surgical margins, in 72% with MMS and 92% with surgical excision after one attempt; 94% of cases eradicated the tumor within two stages.[67] MMS and surgical excision resulted in comparable defects in size on most locations, but defects were more often smaller after MMS only in recurrent tumors on the nose. However, in this study, the cases were not distributed randomly and high-risk tumors were mostly included in the MMS group. When statistical analysis was adjusted for localization and primary and recurrent tumor, it was shown that MMS resulted in smaller defects.[67] Muller and colleagues[68] primarily aimed to compare defect sizes in a randomized prospective study in which low-risk, less than 1 cm in diameter, nodular BCCs were included. The size of final defects after tumor-free margins obtained using 4-mm margins for surgical excision and 2-mm margin for each stage of MMS were compared. This study showed that MMS resulted in smaller defects than surgical excision. All of these studies prove that MMS is superior to surgical excision. Therefore, the procedure of MMS is recommended to avoid large defects for the surgical treatment of NMSCs on the face where the tissue-sparing is very important regarding function and cosmesis, especially for recurrent tumors or tumors with infiltrative aggressive growth pattern.

Complications
The most common complications of surgical treatment of NMSCs are infections, necrosis of grafts and flaps, postoperative bleeding, or a combinations of these.[66] Surgical excision and MMS of primary BBCs did not differ regarding postoperative complications; however, comparisons of complications after the surgical treatment of recurrent BBCs revealed that more complications occurred after surgical excision than after MSS.[66] Esthetic outcomes did not differ between surgical excision and MMS.[66]

Costs
The cost of a treatment option is critical, especially when the affectivity of two treatments is almost equal. Operative costs for a primary BCC were calculated to be $272.11 for surgical excision and $509.18 for MMS; for a recurrent BCC costs increased to $405.93 and $613.69 for surgical excision and MMS, respectively.[66] Higher cost of MMS mainly accounted for higher staff costs because of longer operation times compared with surgical excision.[66] As the lesion size increases, the cost of Mohs surgery becomes much closer to the excision costs.[69] Mohs surgery is estimated to be about 25% more expensive than excision with immediate repair and only 8% more expensive than excision with delayed repair in a cost analysis model.[70] Cook and Zitelli calculated MMS to be 6% more expensive than office excision with permanent sections and 12% and 27% less expensive, respectively, than office excision with frozen sections and ambulatory surgical facility excision on head and neck.[71] Seidler and colleagues[72] estimated MMS in the treatment of facial NMSCs to be less costly and more effective compared with surgical excision in a computer-simulation model. On the contrary, in another study the comparison of cost effectiveness of surgical excision and MMS revealed that MMS was not cost-effective enough to recommend on a large scale for primary and recurrent BCCs, when 30 months' follow-up was considered.[73] However, because of the possibility of increase in recurrence in a longer follow-up period, they also propounded that MMS might become a more cost-effective treatment option for recurrent BCCs.

Management of Incomplete Excision

The incomplete resection rate of NMSCs ranges from 3.2% to 15% for BCCs[2,12,33,34,74–79] and 6.3% to 30.25% for SCC.[12,80,81] Rate of incomplete excision is almost twice more in cases with SCC.[12] Variables most likely to affect the incidence of incomplete excision are as follows:

- Histologic subtype[24,66,74,75,77]
- Anatomic site[12,74,76]
- Size of lesion[12]
- Excision margin[24]
- Multiple synchronous excisions[74,76]
- Grade of surgeon[24,75]

Invasive, morpheic, ulcerative, and multifocal histologic subtypes of BCC are most commonly incompletely excised.[74,77]

The site of the lesion is clearly a major factor influencing the likelihood of an incomplete resection in NMSCs.[12] Because of performing smaller excision to spare skin with cosmetic concerns, incomplete excisions most commonly occur in the midface region. The most common sites where incomplete excisions are seen, are nose, periorbital region, periauricular region, nasolabial fold, cheek, and chin.[12,34,74–76] The rate of incomplete excision of SCC was highest for ear at 20.5%.[81] Cosmetic and functional implications of these areas probably led surgeons to be more conservative to save some crucial structures and to avoid complicated reconstructions.

Recurrence rates of incompletely excised NMSCs have been reported to be between 0% and 27%.[1,35,76,77,82,83] Kyrgidis and colleagues[14] found a correlation between recurrence and positive margins, and there was four-fold increased risk for recurrence when excision margins were positive. Recurrence rate of BCC located on the face was 14.7% in incompletely excised tumors, whereas it was 2.3% in patients with clear margins.[1] When a BCC was excised with positive margins, 21% of observed cases recurred after 5 to 76 months, whereas none of the reoperated cases recurred.[76] Another study found the recurrence rate in patients who were observed to be 25%, whereas it was reduced to 14.3% when immediate re-excision was performed.[77]

Excision of an NMSC with a positive margin does not imply the persistence of tumor. Re-excisions of BCCs with initial positive margins reveal residual tumor in 38.3% to 69.4% of cases.[75,76,78,84] The wide range of negative residual tumor incidence may result from several factors, but the location of the lesion and the biopsy technique were found to be two independent predictors for the negative re-excisions; initially, positive margin located on the face and punch and excisional biopsies reveal more negative re-excisions.[84] Most commonly lateral margins are involved (almost 70%); deep margin and both deep and lateral margin involvement follows.[12,74,75,77] Positivity of lateral margins is more associated with absence of residual tumor in the re-excised lesion, whereas the presence of lateral and deep positive margins may indicate a higher risk of identifying residual BCC in the re-excised lesion.[78]

Management of incompletely excised NMSCs, particularly BCC, is controversial. Because not all incompletely excised BCCs recur, some surgeons strongly recommend immediate re-excision,[66,67] and some propose observation as an option.[38,78,82,83] Smeets and colleagues[66] advocate immediate re-excision, because recurrences lead to larger defects and higher recurrence rates in addition to more aggressiveness. Previously recurrent tumors have larger size and more subclinical extension than primary tumors; therefore, they require more levels of excision and result in a larger defect.[59] On the contrary, Fernandes and colleagues[78] proposed that re-excision is not always necessary when histopathologic positive margin is found in BCC lesions, unless it is high-risk BCC, because nearly two-thirds of the lesions that were submitted to re-excision demonstrated no residual tumor. Hallock and Lutz[82] designed a prospective study to inspect the significance of positive margins regarding recurrence. Recurrence occurred in 13.3% of SCCs with positive margins, but was not seen in patients with BCC, supporting that NMSCs that are not treated do not necessarily recur.

For the management of incompletely excised BCCs of the head and neck, Wilson and colleagues[76] recommended further excision or radiotherapy for all incomplete excisions when local flaps or Wolfe grafts have been used, unless the patient's preference is otherwise; they strongly recommend further excision or radiotherapy when there is involvement of deep-margins in high-risk sites; lateral margin involvement does not rule out the option of observation every 6 months. Rios-Buceta[85] suggests a wait-and-see approach in small primary BCCs that have positive margins, occur at sites other than ears and center of the face, have a nodular or superficial histology, and in elderly patients with multiple complaints or a short life expectancy. Decision making in the management of positive margin involvement without neglecting any of the options including observation, re-excision, or radiotherapy seems more rational. The most appropriate treatment option may be chosen according to general health status of the patient; life expectancy; necessity of challenging reconstructions or loss of functionally and cosmetically crucial structures in case of re-excision or recurrences; patient's preference; and the clinical and the pathologic risk factors of tumor, such as location on high-risk area, tumor greater than 2 cm in diameter, aggressive histopathologic subtype, and recurrent tumor (**Box 2**).

Bovill and colleagues[80] performed a retrospective study to evaluate the clinical and histologic findings in patients with incompletely excised SCC. Re-excisions of incompletely excised SCCs on head and neck contained tumor cells in 31% of specimens. However, the rate of residual tumor in incomplete excision of ear and nose was higher, 58% and 67%, respectively. Macroscopic tumor diameter and Breslow thickness independently contributed to residual SCC. Positive re-excisions were significantly associated with larger tumors, compared with negative re-excisions.

In the management of incompletely excised SCCs, re-excision with a wider margin and deeper plane is the best option.[80,81] Incomplete excision rate of SCC was significantly higher in re-excision of previously incompletely excised lesions than primary excisions.[81] Therefore, treatment of incompletely excised margins of SCC needs great care and experience in the second attempt. Wait-and-see is not a recommended option; when re-excision is not appropriate, radiotherapy provides excellent control without compromising function.[86]

Box 2
Management of incompletely excised NMSCs

Consider re-excision
- If there is deep and lateral margin involvement
- In case of aggressive/infiltrative subtype of BCC
- For any SCCs
- For larger tumors
- Tumors located on high-risk areas
- For young patients
- If there is other clinical and histopathologic risk factors

Wait-and-see approach may be considered
- If there is only lateral margin involvement
- For nodular, superficial BCCs
- For smaller tumors (<1 cm)
- For elderly patients
- If re-excision will lead to loss of function and cosmesis
- If it is patient's preference

REFERENCES

1. Ocanha JP, Dias JT, Miot HA, et al. Relapses and recurrences of basal cell face carcinomas. An Bras Dermatol 2011;86:386–8.
2. Griffiths RW, Suvarna SK, Stone J. Do basal cell carcinomas recur after complete conventional surgical excision? Br J Plast Surg 2005;58:795–805.
3. Batra RS, Kelley LC. A risk scale for predicting extensive subclinical spread of nonmelanoma skin cancer. Dermatol Surg 2002;28:107–12 [discussion: 112].
4. Leibovitch I, Huilgol SC, Selva D, et al. Cutaneous squamous cell carcinoma treated with Mohs micrographic surgery in Australia I. Experience over 10 years. J Am Acad Dermatol 2005;53:253–60.
5. Leibovitch I, Huilgol SC, Selva D, et al. Basal cell carcinoma treated with Mohs surgery in Australia II. Outcome at 5-year follow-up. J Am Acad Dermatol 2005;53:452–7.
6. Swanson NA. Mohs surgery. Technique, indications, applications, and the future. Arch Dermatol 1983; 119:761–73.
7. Veness MJ. High-risk cutaneous squamous cell carcinoma of the head and neck. J Biomed Biotechnol 2007;2007:80572.
8. Takenouchi T, Nomoto S, Ito M. Factors influencing the linear depth of invasion of primary basal cell carcinoma. Dermatol Surg 2001;27:393–6.
9. Silverman MK, Kopf AW, Grin CM, et al. Recurrence rates of treated basal cell carcinomas. Part 2: curettage-electrodesiccation. J Dermatol Surg Oncol 1991;17:720–6.
10. Clayman GL, Lee JJ, Holsinger FC, et al. Mortality risk from squamous cell skin cancer. J Clin Oncol 2005;23:759–65.
11. Mullen JT, Feng L, Xing Y, et al. Invasive squamous cell carcinoma of the skin: defining a high-risk group. Ann Surg Oncol 2006;13:902–9.
12. Bhatti AZ, Asif S, Alwan M. Factors affecting incomplete excision of nonmelanoma skin cancers in New Zealand. Ann Plast Surg 2006;57:513–6.
13. Cherpelis BS, Marcusen C, Lang PG. Prognostic factors for metastasis in squamous cell carcinoma of the skin. Dermatol Surg 2002;28:268–73.
14. Kyrgidis A, Vahtsevanos K, Tzellos TG, et al. Clinical, histological and demographic predictors for recurrence and second primary tumours of head and neck basal cell carcinoma. A 1062 patient-cohort study from a tertiary cancer referral hospital. Eur J Dermatol 2010;20:276–82.
15. McGuire JF, Ge NN, Dyson S. Nonmelanoma skin cancer of the head and neck I: histopathology and clinical behavior. Am J Otolaryngol 2009;30:121–33.

16. Auw-Haedrich C, Frick S, Boehringer D, et al. Histologic safety margin in basal cell carcinoma of the eyelid: correlation with recurrence rate. Ophthalmology 2009;116:802–6.

17. Brantsch KD, Meisner C, Schonfisch B, et al. Analysis of risk factors determining prognosis of cutaneous squamous-cell carcinoma: a prospective study. Lancet Oncol 2008;9:713–20.

18. Cassarino DS, Derienzo DP, Barr RJ. Cutaneous squamous cell carcinoma: a comprehensive clinicopathologic classification. Part one. J Cutan Pathol 2006;33:191–206.

19. Jensen V, Prasad AR, Smith A, et al. Prognostic criteria for squamous cell cancer of the skin. J Surg Res 2010;159:509–16.

20. Kyrgidis A, Tzellos TG, Kechagias N, et al. Cutaneous squamous cell carcinoma (SCC) of the head and neck: risk factors of overall and recurrence-free survival. Eur J Cancer 2010;46:1563–72.

21. Zavos G, Karidis NP, Tsourouflis G, et al. Nonmelanoma skin cancer after renal transplantation: a single-center experience in 1736 transplantations. Int J Dermatol 2011;50:1496–500.

22. Lott DG, Manz R, Koch C, et al. Aggressive behavior of nonmelanotic skin cancers in solid organ transplant recipients. Transplantation 2010;90:683–7.

23. Harwood CA, Proby CM, McGregor JM, et al. Clinicopathologic features of skin cancer in organ transplant recipients: a retrospective case-control series. J Am Acad Dermatol 2006;54:290–300.

24. Kumar P, Watson S, Brain AN, et al. Incomplete excision of basal cell carcinoma: a prospective multicentre audit. Br J Plast Surg 2002;55:616–22.

25. Carducci M, Bozzetti M, de Marco G, et al. Preoperative margin detection by digital dermoscopy in the traditional surgical excision of cutaneous squamous cell carcinomas. J Dermatolog Treat 2012. http://dx.doi.org/10.3109/09546634.2012.672711.

26. Carducci M, Bozzetti M, de Marco G, et al. Usefulness of margin detection by digital dermoscopy in the traditional surgical excision of basal cell carcinomas of the head and neck including infiltrative/morpheaform type. J Dermatol 2012;39(4):326–30.

27. Caresana G, Giardini R. Dermoscopy-guided surgery in basal cell carcinoma. J Eur Acad Dermatol Venereol 2010;24:1395–9.

28. Chiller K, Passaro D, McCalmont T, et al. Efficacy of curettage before excision in clearing surgical margins of nonmelanoma skin cancer. Arch Dermatol 2000;136:1327–32.

29. Ghosh S, Duvvi S, Goodyear P, et al. Evaluation of surgeons' marking of excision margins for superficial facial skin cancer lesions. J Laryngol Otol 2009;123:195–8.

30. Wettstein R, Kalbermatten DF, Rieger U, et al. High magnification assessment improves complete resection of facial tumors. Ann Plast Surg 2006;57:517–20.

31. Wolf DJ, Zitelli JA. Surgical margins for basal cell carcinoma. Arch Dermatol 1987;123:340–4.

32. Kimyai-Asadi A, Alam M, Goldberg LH, et al. Efficacy of narrow-margin excision of well-demarcated primary facial basal cell carcinomas. J Am Acad Dermatol 2005;53:464–8.

33. Bisson MA, Dunkin CS, Suvarna SK, et al. Do plastic surgeons resect basal cell carcinomas too widely? A prospective study comparing surgical and histological margins. Br J Plast Surg 2002;55:293–7.

34. Griffiths RW, Suvarna SK, Stone J. Basal cell carcinoma histological clearance margins: an analysis of 1539 conventionally excised tumours. Wider still and deeper? J Plast Reconstr Aesthet Surg 2007;60:41–7.

35. Gulleth Y, Goldberg N, Silverman RP, et al. What is the best surgical margin for a basal cell carcinoma: a meta-analysis of the literature. Plast Reconstr Surg 2010;126:1222–31.

36. Brodland DG, Zitelli JA. Surgical margins for excision of primary cutaneous squamous cell carcinoma. J Am Acad Dermatol 1992;27:241–8.

37. Thomas DJ, King AR, Peat BG. Excision margins for nonmelanotic skin cancer. Plast Reconstr Surg 2003;112:57–63.

38. Unlu RE, Altun S, Kerem M, et al. Is it really necessary to make wide excisions for basal cell carcinoma treatment? J Craniofac Surg 2009;20:1989–91.

39. Smith-Zagone MJ, Schwartz MR. Frozen section of skin specimens. Arch Pathol Lab Med 2005;129:1536–43.

40. Lane JE, Kent DE. Surgical margins in the treatment of nonmelanoma skin cancer and Mohs micrographic surgery. Curr Surg 2005;62:518–26.

41. Ghauri RR, Gunter AA, Weber RA. Frozen section analysis in the management of skin cancers. Ann Plast Surg 1999;43:156–60.

42. Manstein ME, Manstein CH, Smith R. How accurate is frozen section for skin cancers? Ann Plast Surg 2003;50:607–9.

43. Bogdanov-Berezovsky A, Rosenberg L, Cagniano E, et al. The role of frozen section histological analysis in the treatment of head and neck skin basal and squamous cell carcinomas. Isr Med Assoc J 2008;10:344–5.

44. Kimyai-Asadi A, Goldberg LH, Jih MH. Accuracy of serial transverse cross-sections in detecting residual basal cell carcinoma at the surgical margins of an elliptical excision specimen. J Am Acad Dermatol 2005;53:469–74.

45. Niederhagen B, von Lindern JJ, Berge S, et al. Staged operations for basal cell carcinoma of the face. Br J Oral Maxillofac Surg 2000;38:477–9.

46. Hsuan JD, Harrad RA, Potts MJ, et al. Small margin excision of periocular basal cell carcinoma: 5 year results. Br J Ophthalmol 2004;88:358–60.

47. Eskiizmir G, Gencoglan G, Temiz P, et al. Staged-surgery with permanent pathology for the management of high-risk nonmelanoma skin cancer of the nose. Eur Arch Otorhinolaryngol 2011;268:117–21.

48. Goto M, Kai Y, Arakawa S, et al. Analysis of 256 cases of basal cell carcinoma after either one-step or two-step surgery in a Japanese institution. J Dermatol 2012;39:68–71.

49. Hafner HM, Breuninger H, Moehrle M, et al. 3D histology-guided surgery for basal cell carcinoma and squamous cell carcinoma: recurrence rates and clinical outcome. Int J Oral Maxillofac Surg 2011;40:943–8.

50. Trost LB, Bailin PL. History of Mohs surgery. Dermatol Clin 2011;29:135–9, vii.

51. Ratner D, Bagiella E. The efficacy of curettage in delineating margins of basal cell carcinoma before Mohs micrographic surgery. Dermatol Surg 2003; 29:899–903.

52. Chung VQ, Bernardo L, Jiang SB. Presurgical curettage appropriately reduces the number of Mohs stages by better delineating the subclinical extensions of tumor margins. Dermatol Surg 2005;31: 1094–9 [discussion: 1100].

53. Jih MH, Friedman PM, Goldberg LH, et al. Curettage prior to Mohs' micrographic surgery for previously biopsied nonmelanoma skin cancers: what are we curetting? Retrospective, prospective, and comparative study. Dermatol Surg 2005;31:10–5.

54. Huang CC, Boyce S, Northington M, et al. Randomized, controlled surgical trial of preoperative tumor curettage of basal cell carcinoma in Mohs micrographic surgery. J Am Acad Dermatol 2004;51: 585–91.

55. Bagheri S, King T, Justiniano H, et al. Maintaining tissue orientation during Mohs micrographic surgery: scalpel versus marker. Dermatol Surg 2011;37:1412–6.

56. Benedetto PX, Poblete-Lopez C. Mohs micrographic surgery technique. Dermatol Clin 2011;29:141–51, vii.

57. Gurgen J, Judy D, Witfill K, et al. An alternative approach for Mohs surgery using a combination of a flexible blade and the traditional scalpel. J Eur Acad Dermatol Venereol 2011. http://dx.doi.org/ 10.1111/j.1468–3083.2011.04341.x.

58. Campbell RM, Barrall D, Wilkel C, et al. Post-Mohs micrographic surgical margin tissue evaluation with permanent histopathologic sections. Dermatol Surg 2005;31:655–8 [discussion: 658].

59. Leibovitch I, Huilgol SC, Selva D, et al. Basal cell carcinoma treated with Mohs surgery in Australia I. Experience over 10 years. J Am Acad Dermatol 2005;53:445–51.

60. Orengo IF, Salasche SJ, Fewkes J, et al. Correlation of histologic subtypes of primary basal cell carcinoma and number of Mohs stages required to achieve a tumor-free plane. J Am Acad Dermatol 1997;37:395–7.

61. Smeets NW, Kuijpers DI, Nelemans P, et al. Mohs' micrographic surgery for treatment of basal cell carcinoma of the face–results of a retrospective study and review of the literature. Br J Dermatol 2004;151:141–7.

62. Mosterd K, Krekels GA, Nieman FH, et al. Surgical excision versus Mohs' micrographic surgery for primary and recurrent basal-cell carcinoma of the face: a prospective randomised controlled trial with 5-years' follow-up. Lancet Oncol 2008;9:1149–56.

63. Asgari MM, Warton EM, Neugebauer R, et al. Predictors of patient satisfaction with Mohs surgery: analysis of preoperative, intraoperative, and postoperative factors in a prospective cohort. Arch Dermatol 2011;147:1387–94.

64. Paoli J, Daryoni S, Wennberg AM, et al. 5-year recurrence rates of Mohs micrographic surgery for aggressive and recurrent facial basal cell carcinoma. Acta Derm Venereol 2011;91:689–93.

65. Chren MM, Torres JS, Stuart SE, et al. Recurrence after treatment of nonmelanoma skin cancer: a prospective cohort study. Arch Dermatol 2011; 147:540–6.

66. Smeets NW, Krekels GA, Ostertag JU, et al. Surgical excision vs Mohs' micrographic surgery for basal-cell carcinoma of the face: randomised controlled trial. Lancet 2004;364:1766–72.

67. Van der Eerden PA, Prins ME, Lohuis PJ, et al. Eighteen years of experience in Mohs micrographic surgery and conventional excision for nonmelanoma skin cancer treated by a single facial plastic surgeon and pathologist. Laryngoscope 2010;120: 2378–84.

68. Muller FM, Dawe RS, Moseley H, et al. Randomized comparison of Mohs micrographic surgery and surgical excision for small nodular basal cell carcinoma: tissue-sparing outcome. Dermatol Surg 2009;35:1349–54.

69. Holmkvist KA, Rogers GS, Dahl PR. Incidence of residual basal cell carcinoma in patients who appear tumor free after biopsy. J Am Acad Dermatol 1999;41:600–5.

70. Rogers HW, Coldiron BM. A relative value unit-based cost comparison of treatment modalities for nonmelanoma skin cancer: effect of the loss of the Mohs multiple surgery reduction exemption. J Am Acad Dermatol 2009;61:96–103.

71. Cook J, Zitelli JA. Mohs micrographic surgery: a cost analysis. J Am Acad Dermatol 1998;39: 698–703.

72. Seidler AM, Bramlette TB, Washington CV, et al. Mohs versus traditional surgical excision for facial and auricular nonmelanoma skin cancer: an analysis of cost-effectiveness. Dermatol Surg 2009;35: 1776–87.

73. Essers BA, Dirksen CD, Nieman FH, et al. Cost-effectiveness of Mohs micrographic surgery vs surgical excision for basal cell carcinoma of the face. Arch Dermatol 2006;142:187–94.

74. Farhi D, Dupin N, Palangie A, et al. Incomplete excision of basal cell carcinoma: rate and associated factors among 362 consecutive cases. Dermatol Surg 2007;33:1207–14.

75. Malik V, Goh KS, Leong S, et al. Risk and outcome analysis of 1832 consecutively excised basal cell carcinomas in a tertiary referral plastic surgery unit. J Plast Reconstr Aesthet Surg 2010;63:2057–63.

76. Wilson AW, Howsam G, Santhanam V, et al. Surgical management of incompletely excised basal cell carcinomas of the head and neck. Br J Oral Maxillofac Surg 2004;42:311–4.

77. Sherry KR, Reid LA, Wilmshurst AD. A five year review of basal cell carcinoma excisions. J Plast Reconstr Aesthet Surg 2010;63:1485–9.

78. Fernandes JD, de Lorenzo Messina MC, de Almeida Pimentel ER, et al. Presence of residual basal cell carcinoma in re-excised specimens is more probable when deep and lateral margins were positive. J Eur Acad Dermatol Venereol 2008;22:704–6.

79. Santiago F, Serra D, Vieira R, et al. Incidence and factors associated with recurrence after incomplete excision of basal cell carcinomas: a study of 90 cases. J Eur Acad Dermatol Venereol 2010;24:1421–4.

80. Bovill ES, Cullen KW, Barrett W, et al. Clinical and histological findings in re-excision of incompletely excised cutaneous squamous cell carcinoma. J Plast Reconstr Aesthet Surg 2009;62:457–61.

81. Tan PY, Ek E, Su S, et al. Incomplete excision of squamous cell carcinoma of the skin: a prospective observational study. Plast Reconstr Surg 2007;120:910–6.

82. Hallock GG, Lutz DA. A prospective study of the accuracy of the surgeon's diagnosis and significance of positive margins in nonmelanoma skin cancers. Plast Reconstr Surg 2001;107:942–7.

83. Rieger KE, Linos E, Egbert BM. Recurrence rates associated with incompletely excised low-risk nonmelanoma skin cancer. J Cutan Pathol 2010;37:59–67.

84. Macpherson N, Lamrock E, Watt G. Effect of inflammation on positive margins of basal cell carcinomas. Australas J Dermatol 2010;51:95–8.

85. Rios-Buceta L. Management of basal cell carcinomas with positive margins. Actas Dermosifiliogr 2007;98:679–87 [in Spanish].

86. Veness MJ. Treatment recommendations in patients diagnosed with high-risk cutaneous squamous cell carcinoma. Australas Radiol 2005;49:365–76.

Cutaneous Squamous Cell Carcinoma of the Head and Neck
Management of the Parotid and Neck

Metin Yilmaz, MD[a],*, Görkem Eskiizmir, MD[b],
Oren Friedman, MD[c]

KEYWORDS

- Cutaneous squamous cell carcinoma • Metastasis • Parotid • Neck

KEY POINTS

- There are certain characteristics to a primary lesion of cutaneous squamous cell carcinoma (SCC) that imply a higher risk of lymphatic metastasis, such as size, thickness, and histopathologic features (differentiation, perineural involvement, desmoplasia, and so forth).
- The presence of lymph node disease is a poor prognostic factor in cutaneous SCC.
- Cutaneous SCC of the head and neck can spread to parotid lymph nodes, cervical lymph nodes, or both, depending on the location of the primary tumor. Therefore, clinical and radiologic evaluation of the parotid and neck should be performed in patients with cutaneous SCC.
- The optimal treatment for metastatic cutaneous SCC of the head and neck should be complete surgical resection with adjuvant radiotherapy.

INTRODUCTION

Skin cancer is the most common malignancy in the white population, and is related to chronic solar ultraviolet radiation.[1] Although the head and neck comprises only 9% of the total body surface area, most nonmelanoma skin cancers are encountered in this region as a result of sun exposure. The incidence of cutaneous squamous cell carcinoma (SCC) of the head and neck accounts for approximately 20% to 25% of all nonmelanoma skin cancers.[1–4] Cutaneous SCC of the head and neck rarely metastasizes to regional lymph nodes (approximately 5% of patients), but when it does the parotid lymph node bed is most frequently involved.[2,5] Patients with metastatic cutaneous SCC have a poor prognosis with an overall 5-year survival rate of 34.4%.[6] Therefore, the detection of macrometastasis or micrometastasis of parotid and/or cervical lymph nodes is crucial. Because the involvement of lymph nodes in cutaneous SCC of the head and neck is relatively uncommon, and as it often takes a long time from the initial tumor identification and treatment to the ultimate development of metastases, it is worthwhile highlighting the disease process to bring it to the forefront of the clinician's mind. The aim of this article is to review the lymphatic drainage of skin, the principles of lymphatic metastasis, risk factors and patterns of tumor spread, and the staging and therapeutic implications of metastatic cutaneous SCC of the head and neck.

[a] Department of Otolaryngology-Head and Neck Surgery, Gazi University Hospital, Beşevler, Ankara, Turkey;
[b] Department of Otolaryngology-Head and Neck Surgery, Celal Bayar University, Uncubozköy yerleşkesi, 45030, Manisa, Turkey; [c] Facial Plastic Surgery, Otolaryngology-Head and Neck Surgery, University of Pennsylvania, Philadelphia, PA, USA
* Corresponding author.
E-mail address: drmyilmaz@gazi.edu.tr

Facial Plast Surg Clin N Am 20 (2012) 473–481
http://dx.doi.org/10.1016/j.fsc.2012.07.007

CUTANEOUS LYMPHATIC SYSTEM OF THE HEAD AND NECK

The lymphatic system is an important component of the immune system, playing a vital role in infection, inflammation, and cancer metastasis. It provides a pathway for the drainage of lymph, a white, "milky" fluid that contains proteins, lipids, cells, cellular debris, and foreign products. The lymphatic system includes a terminal capillary network, precollector and collector lymph vessels, lymphatic ducts, and lymph nodes. The superficial lymphatic plexus is located in the upper dermis (near the arterial plexus) and collects lymph from the interstitium. Lymphatic capillaries have an endothelial leaflet layer, and an incomplete basement membrane and muscle layer; however, they do not have intraluminal valves.[7,8] These capillaries are generally tortuous, and several lymphatic capillaries join in the dermis to form lymphatic vessels called precollectors. Precollector lymphatic vessels have a complete endothelial layer, basement membrane, and muscle layer with intraluminal valves, which are separated by approximately 2-mm intervals.[9] Thereafter, lymphatic fluid enters collector lymphatic vessels at the cutis-subcutis boundary. The collector lymphatic vessels have a continuous basal membrane, valves, and smooth muscle cells, which play a vital role in lymph transport by propelling lymph toward afferent vessels that ultimately drain into lymph nodes. Thus, unidirectional lymph flow in lymphatic vessels is maintained by an intrinsic pump mechanism, and retrograde lymph flow is prevented by internal valves. The velocity of lymph flow is variable throughout the body and is relatively slow in the head and neck (approximately 1.5 cm/min).[10]

In the head and neck region there are more than 300 lymph nodes, subclassified into lymph node groups. Lymph node groups are generally named according to their locations: suboccipital, retroauricular, parotid, facial (buccal), retropharyngeal, and cervical (submental, submandibular, upper jugular, middle jugular, lower jugular, anterior jugular, spinal accessory chain, and supraclavicular). The patterns of lymphatic drainage in the head and neck are categorized as follows[11]:

1. Main lymphatic pathway: drains anterior face, oral cavity, and nasal mucosa
2. Posterior accessory lymphatic pathway: drains the postauricular region, posterior scalp, suboccipital region, nasopharynx, and oropharynx
3. Anterior lymphatic pathway: drains the oral cavity, median part of the lower lip, and the skin overlying the chin
4. Superficial lateral pathway: drains the posterior scalp and initially enters the suboccipital and retroauricular nodes

The lymphatic drainage pathways for the skin of the head and neck region are usually predictable, and are presented in **Table 1**.[12,13]

The parotid gland has a high-density lymphatic network. It has been demonstrated that intraparotid lymph nodes are "trafficking" the lymphatic metastasis of cutaneous SCC, in particular for tumors located on the lateral part of the face (**Fig. 1**).[14] Marks[15] dissected 1 to 11 lymph nodes from the parotid gland in a series of 17 radical parotidectomies. He found that on average, one node remains in the deep lobe of the parotid following superficial parotidectomy. Similarly, McKean and colleagues[16] found that almost all lymph nodes of the parotid gland are located lateral to the facial nerve, in the so-called superficial lobe of the gland.

LYMPHATIC METASTASIS OF CUTANEOUS SCC OF THE HEAD AND NECK

Lymphatic metastasis is one of the major determinants in the staging, treatment, and prognosis of head and neck malignancies. Lymphatic

Table 1	
Lymphatic drainage of skin in the head and neck	
Anatomic Region	**Lymph Node Group**
Eyelid and eyebrows	Parotid, submandibular
Anterior ear and preauricular region	Parotid
Helix and lateral aspect of the auricle	Retroauricular, suboccipital
Cheek, nose, upper lip	Parotid, submandibular
Lateral part of lower lip	Submandibular
Median lower lip, chin	Submental
Lateral aspect of the head and forehead	Parotid, upper jugulodigastric
Frontal and parietal parts of scalp	Parotid
Posterior part of scalp and head	Suboccipital, retroauricular, upper, middle and lower jugulodigastric, supraclavicular
Neck	Upper, middle, and lower jugulodigastric

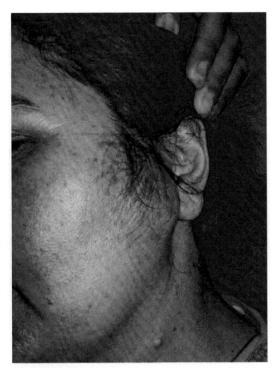

Fig. 1. A patient who was referred because of involvement of parotid lymph nodes following surgical resection of cutaneous SCC of the face.

metastasis is generally initiated when the tumor directly penetrates the basement membrane of the epithelium and invades the extracellular matrix. This process is facilitated by the impairment of adhesive properties of tumor cells, secretion of proteolytic enzymes, and increase in intratumoral interstitial fluid pressure. Tumor cells enter the lymph through peritumoral and intratumoral lymphatic capillaries, which are dilated and hyperplastic, by means of hydrostatic pressure gradients and active movement. The development and proliferation of peritumoral and intratumoral lymphatic capillaries are triggered by lymphangiogenesis, which is mediated by growth factors, cytokines, and chemokines mainly secreted from tumor cells and/or host cells.[17,18] Recent studies have demonstrated that the vascular endothelial growth factor (VEGF)-C/VEGF-D/VEGF receptor-3 signaling axis plays a vital role in lymphangiogenesis, and promotes formation of tumor lymphatics and metastatic spread of tumor cells to lymph nodes.[19–23] Vascular endothelial growth factor-C and/or VEGF-D expression in tumor cells stimulates VEGF receptor-3, a cell-surface receptor tyrosine kinase located on lymphatic endothelial cells, and activates growth of lymphatic vessels. In addition, VEGF-A, platelet-derived growth factor BB, and hepatocyte growth factor have been linked to lymphangiogenesis and

lymphatic metastasis.[24,25] Finally, tumor cells are transported to the subscapular sinus of lymph node via lymphatic vessels. Unfortunately, lymph nodes are poor barriers for tumor spread. Therefore, only small numbers of tumor cells are destroyed while most tumor cells can easily settle and proliferate in the subscapular sinus of the first-echelon lymph node. Further metastasis to other lymph nodes is almost inevitable once the cortex of a sentinel lymph node (SLN) is invaded.

PATIENT WITH HIGH-RISK CUTANEOUS SCC OF THE HEAD AND NECK

Most patients with cutaneous SCC of the head and neck are at low risk of developing local recurrence, lymph node metastasis, and distant metastasis. However, there is a subset of patients who are at high risk for local recurrence and nodal metastasis, and in whom long-term survival is very low. These patients should be carefully evaluated for the presence of macrometastasis or micrometastasis in regional lymph nodes. In such patients, SLN biopsy or elective parotidectomy/neck dissection should be considered, even when lymph node metastasis is not detected on clinical or radiologic evaluation. This high-risk cutaneous SCC patient group is defined by patient-related, tumor-related, and previous treatment–related risk factors (**Table 2**).

Evaluation of the Patient

A complete head and neck examination including a search for lymph node metastasis is required in

---

Table 2
The criteria for high-risk cutaneous SCC of the head and neck

Patient-related factors
Immunocompromised patients (Transplant recipients, leukemia)

Tumor-related factors
Tumor size (>2 cm)
Tumor thickness (>4 mm, Clark level IV and V)
Tumor characteristic (poorly differentiated, Broders' grade 3 and 4)
Tumor location (ear, lip commissure)
Tumor with perineural invasion
Tumor with lymphovascular invasion
Tumor histopathology (Adenoid, adenosquamous, desmoplastic type)
Tumor developing from scar or burn
Recurrent tumor
Rapid growth pattern

Previous treatment-related factors
Incomplete excision
Radiotherapy

all patients, but especially in those with high-risk cutaneous SCC. In addition, radiological evaluation with ultrasonography, computed tomography, or magnetic resonance imaging should be performed for staging, although the diagnostic value of these techniques is controversial in the absence of clinically enlarged lymph nodes. Cho and colleagues[26] retrospectively investigated the role of whole-body ^{18}F-fluorodeoxyglucose (FDG) positron emission tomography (PET) for staging cutaneous SCC, and suggested that ^{18}F-FDG PET can be useful for the assessment of patients with high-risk cutaneous SCC. Ultrasound-guided fine-needle aspiration can also be useful for the detection of occult lymph node metastasis, although limited information can be obtained for micrometastasis and lymph nodes smaller than 4 mm.[27] In addition, SLN biopsy may be a diagnostic option for patients with cutaneous SCC.

Sentinel lymph nodes are defined as the first-echelon lymph nodes that receive lymph drainage directly from a tumor site; thus these lymph nodes, theoretically, have the highest risk of having lymphatic metastasis. The theory behind SLN biopsy is that SLNs should be strong predictors of lymphatic metastasis by demonstrating the presence or absence of metastatic disease. Sentinel node biopsies are generally performed using ^{99}Tc-labeled colloid radiotracer and/or a dye such as methylene blue. This technique is a widely accepted modality in managing breast cancer and melanoma; however, the true clinical value of SLN biopsy in head and neck cancers remains unclear, in part because of the complex lymphatic network.

The evidence to date regarding the diagnostic value of SLN biopsy in cutaneous SCC of the head and neck is inconclusive. In 2006, Ross and Schmults[28] reviewed the literature and found a total of 692 cutaneous SCC patients who underwent SLN biopsy. Of these, only 85 cases were nonanogenital (the exact number of patients with head and neck involvement was not stated). Ross and Schmults emphasized that SLN biopsy in high-risk cutaneous SCC is an emerging diagnostic technique. However, prospective, randomized, clinical studies of larger populations are required to assess its clinical applicability and utility.

Staging Systems: Cutaneous SCC of the Head and Neck

A validated, standard, and accurate staging system is vital for all malignancies to reflect the extent of disease, predict the prognosis, and determine the ideal treatment modality. At present, three different nodal staging systems have been designed for cutaneous SCC (**Table 3**):

Table 3
Nodal staging systems of cutaneous SCC of the head and neck

TNM classification (American Joint Committee on Cancer, 2010)	
N0	No regional lymph node metastasis
N1	Single ipsilateral lymph node metastasis, maximal diameter <3 cm
N2a	Single ipsilateral lymph node metastasis, maximal diameter >3 cm to maximum 6 cm
N2b	Multiple ipsilateral lymph node metastasis, all with maximal diameter ≤6 cm
N2c	Multiple bilateral or contralateral lymph node metastasis, all with maximal diameter ≤6
N3	Lymph node metastasis with diameter >6 cm
O'Brien P/N classification	
Parotid	
P0	No clinical disease in the parotid
P1	Metastatic node up to 3 cm in diameter
P2	Metastatic node >3 cm and up to 6 cm in diameter or multiple nodes
P3	Metastatic node >6 cm or disease involving the facial nerve or skull base
Neck	
N0	No clinical disease
N1	Single ipsilateral neck node up to 3 cm in diameter
N2	Single node >3 cm in diameter or multiple nodes or contralateral nodes
N1S3	
Stage I	Single lymph node <3 cm
Stage II	Single lymph node >3 cm or multiple nodes <3 cm
Stage III	Multiple nodes maximum diameter >3 cm

1. TNM staging system of the American Joint Committee on Cancer (AJCC)
2. O'Brien P/N classification
3. N1S3 staging system

The seventh edition of the AJCC staging manual for cutaneous SCC mainly involves Tumor (designating the location, size, thickness, histopathologic features of primary tumor, and bone, cartilage, and muscle involvement), Node (designating the amount, location, and size of metastatic lymph node disease), and Metastasis (designating the presence of distant metastasis). The N staging system of cutaneous SCC is almost identical to mucosal head and neck SCCs. However, the effectiveness of this staging system for stratification of patients with cutaneous SCC in reflecting the potential risk of lymphatic metastasis and prognosis is unclear. Farasat and colleagues[29] stated that the AJCC staging system provides coordinated, consistent data for assessing the prognosis in cutaneous SCC. On the other hand, Breuninger and colleagues[30] emphasized the deficiencies of this system in clinical applicability and prognostic value.

In 2002, O'Brien and colleagues[31] proposed a staging system, entitled the O'Brien P/N staging system, for patients with cutaneous SCC of the head and neck. It primarily notes the absence/presence, location (parotid and/or neck), size, amount, and invasion (to facial nerve and/or skull base) of lymph nodes. In the proposed staging system, the investigators classified 87 patients with cutaneous SCC of the head and neck. The involvement of lymph nodes in both the parotid gland and neck, larger (larger than 3 cm) nodes, and/or multiple cervical lymph node metastasis were determined as poor prognostic factors; thus, they offered the separation of parotid and neck lymph node disease for the prognostication of cutaneous SCC. Thereafter, Andruchow and colleagues[32] designed a retrospective, multicenter study in which 322 patients with cutaneous SCC of the head and neck were reevaluated and restaged according to the O'Brien P/N staging system. The investigators concluded that separation of parotid and neck lymph node disease is beneficial for staging cutaneous SCC. Hinerman and colleagues[3] also preferred the O'Brien P/N staging system because of its improved prognostication of cutaneous SCC progression.

In 2010 a new staging system for metastatic head and neck cutaneous SCC, referred to as N1S3, was proposed to facilitate a better prognostic discrimination.[33] In this staging system, Forest and colleagues[33] suggested gathering the parotid and neck lymph node groups together instead of separating them as O'Brien P/N had proposed. The N1S3 system stratified the patients based on 2 predictors: the size and amount of metastatic lymph nodes. This staging system was applied to 215 patients with cutaneous SCC, and its predictive capacity for locoregional control, disease-specific survival, and overall survival was found to be remarkably high. However, multicenter, prospective, large-population studies are needed for the validation of this staging system.

Treatment Modalities

The contemporary treatment modality suggested for metastatic cutaneous SCC of the head and neck is surgical resection (parotidectomy, neck dissection, or both) with adjuvant radiotherapy (**Fig. 2**).[34,35] The surgical plan should be tailored according to the involved lymph node groups. In a multicenter clinical trial, Andruchow and colleagues[32] demonstrated a significant dominance of the involvement of parotid lymph nodes (only parotid lymph node in 67%, both parotid and cervical lymph nodes in 13%) in patients with cutaneous SCC of the head and neck. Therefore, the parotid gland is referred to as the metastatic "basin" for cutaneous SCC of the head and neck.[5] The majority of metastatic nodal disease in the parotid gland is located in the superficial lobe; therefore, a superficial parotidectomy with preservation of the facial nerve is the recommended surgical treatment for metastatic cutaneous SCC to the parotid gland. The deep lobe should be evaluated intraoperatively by inspection and palpation, and surgical resection should be extended in cases of suspicion for deep lobe nodal involvement. Every attempt for the preservation of facial nerve should be made during parotidectomy. Iyer and colleagues[36] examined the surgical outcomes in patients who underwent parotidectomy for metastatic disease of cutaneous SCC who had known microscopic residual disease adjacent to the facial nerve postoperatively. The investigators found that performing a facial nerve-sparing parotidectomy and adjuvant radiotherapy in patients who had metastatic cutaneous SCC to the parotid and microscopic residual disease involving the facial nerve after surgery did not portend a worsened prognosis for local recurrence or shorter survival. On occasion, when the nerve is grossly involved or in cases of progressive facial paralysis, resection of the facial nerves is required.[35,37] A comprehensive neck dissection should also be performed concurrently in patients who have clinically positive metastatic disease of both the parotid and cervical nodes (see **Fig. 2**). In addition, adjuvant radiotherapy following surgical resection of nodal disease in the parotid gland and/or neck should be planned to improve overall outcome.[1,38–40]

The incidence of occult metastasis to cervical lymph nodes was reported in 14.7% to 44% of patients who had clinically positive parotid lymph node metastasis.[12,38,41–44] It has been

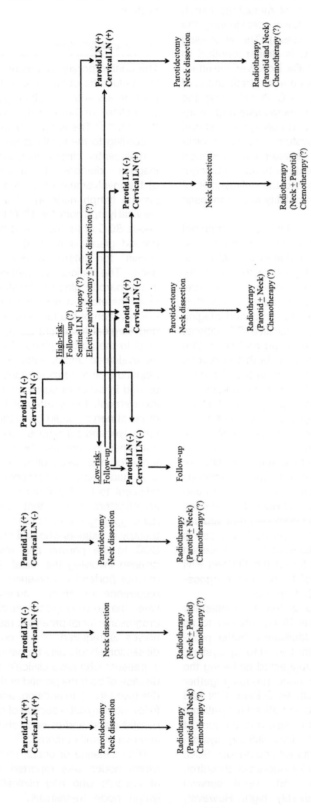

Fig. 2. An algorithmic approach to metastatic cutaneous SCC of the head and neck. LN, lymph node.

demonstrated that level II is the most frequently involved cervical region (79%) among lymph node–positive neck dissections.[12] On the other hand, lymphatic metastasis to level IV and V is rare in most cases. However, in posterior scalp tumors, level V metastases are more common. In a recent clinical trial, 295 neck dissections that were performed for clinically positive regional metastases from cutaneous SCC of the head and neck were analyzed, and involvement of lymph nodes at different levels of the neck were noted and correlated with the site of the primary tumor.[45] It was concluded that level I involvement in the absence of level II or level III involvement can be observed more commonly in patients with midline facial primaries. In addition, the involvement of levels IV and V was analyzed, whereby none of the tumors of the external ear had lymph node metastasis to levels IV or V, and only 2.7% of tumors arising in the face and anterior scalp had lymph node metastasis to levels IV or V. However, the involvement of levels IV and V was significantly higher (15.8%) in patients who had cutaneous SCC located on the posterior scalp and neck. Based on these findings, selective neck dissection including levels I to III is suggested for patients with primary tumors of midline facial structures, selective neck dissection including levels II to III for patients with primary tumors of anterior scalp and external ear, and selective neck dissection including levels II to V for patients with primary tumors of posterior scalp and neck (see **Fig. 2**).[35,45]

The management of patients with clinically N0 cutaneous SCC of the head and neck is controversial (see **Fig. 2**). Of note, a precise clinical evaluation and radiological examination should be performed preoperatively. Recently, SLN biopsy has engendered much interest as a promising diagnostic tool for the identification of occult lymph node metastasis in patients with high-risk cutaneous SCC of the head and neck. A clinical study with a large cohort of patients is required to prove its utility in this patient group. In a retrospective study, the role of elective parotidectomy was evaluated in 19 patients who underwent total auriculectomy and parotidectomy for advanced auricular cutaneous SCC without clinically and radiographically positive lymph nodes in the parotid gland.[46] All parotid specimens were examined histologically, and no signs of occult lymph node metastasis were detected. Therefore, the investigators suggested avoiding elective parotidectomy for patients with advanced auricular cutaneous SCC without clinically and radiographically positive parotid lymph nodes. In a separate study by Yoon and colleagues,[47] a high rate of

local and regional recurrence, and distant metastasis in patients with auricular cutaneous SCC was reported. These investigators suggested aggressive surgical treatment of the primary lesion in addition to treatment of regional lymph nodes, including the parotid gland, for auricular cutaneous SCC. Similarly, Peiffer and colleagues[48] noted a high rate of occult lymph node metastasis in patients with advanced cutaneous SCC, and offered their patients elective lymph node dissection and parotidectomy even in the absence of clinically evident lymph node metastasis. Based on the current clinical evidence, the authors also recommend elective neck dissection and parotidectomy in patients with high-risk cutaneous SCC as defined in **Table 2**.

In the literature there are limited data that demonstrate the efficacy of systemic chemotherapy in the treatment of metastatic cutaneous SCC. However, concurrent chemoradiation is generally offered to patients who have cutaneous SCC of the head and neck with extensive lymph node metastasis, although a standard treatment modality has not yet been formulated.[49] A pilot study from the Peter MacCallum Cancer Institute demonstrated better control of local and regional recurrence with concomitant platinum-based chemotherapy and radiotherapy following surgical resection.[37] In addition, promising outcomes were reported with targeted therapies (tyrosine kinase inhibitors and/or epidermal growth factor receptor [EGFR] inhibitors) in patients with advanced cutaneous SCC. Wollina[50] recently reviewed the efficacy of cetuximab, an EGFR inhibitor, in cutaneous SCC, and emphasized that the combination of radiotherapy with cetuximab seems to have better outcomes in patients with recurrent or advanced cutaneous SCC; however, most of the evidence involves case reports or limited case series. Prospective, randomized rigorous clinical trials are required before establishing the role of chemotherapy in cutaneous SCC.

REFERENCES

1. Veness MJ, Morgan GJ, Palme CE, et al. Surgery and adjuvant radiotherapy in patients with cutaneous head and neck squamous cell carcinoma metastatic to lymph nodes: combined treatment should be considered best practice. Laryngoscope 2005;115:870–5.
2. Ch'ng S, Maitra A, Allison RS, et al. Parotid and cervical nodal status predict prognosis for patients with head and neck metastatic cutaneous squamous cell carcinoma. J Surg Oncol 2008;98:101–5.

3. Hinerman RW, Indelicato DJ, Amdur RJ, et al. Cutaneous squamous cell carcinoma metastatic to parotid-area lymph nodes. Laryngoscope 2008; 118:1989–96.

4. D'Souza J, Clark J. Management of the neck in metastatic cutaneous squamous cell carcinoma of the head and neck. Curr Opin Otolaryngol Head Neck Surg 2011;19:99–105.

5. O'Brien CJ. The parotid gland as a metastatic basin for cutaneous cancer. Arch Otolaryngol Head Neck Surg 2005;131:551–5.

6. Rowe DE, Carroll RJ, Day CL. Prognostic factors for local recurrence, metastasis, and survival rates in squamous cell carcinoma of the skin, ear, and lip. J Am Acad Dermatol 1992;26:976–90.

7. Feely MA, Olsen KD, Gamble GL, et al. Cutaneous lymphatics and chronic lymphedema of the head and neck. Clin Anat 2012;25:72–85.

8. Uren RF, Howman-Giles R, Thompson JF. Patterns of lymphatic drainage from the skin in patients with melanoma. J Nucl Med 2003;44:570–82.

9. Pan WR, le Roux CM, Levy SM, et al. The morphology of the human lymphatic vessels in the head and neck. Clin Anat 2010;23:654–61.

10. Uren RF. Lymphatic drainage of the skin. Ann Surg Oncol 2004;11:179S–85S.

11. Lengelé B, Hamoir M, Scalliet P, et al. Anatomical bases for the radiological delineation of lymph node areas. Major collecting trunks, head and neck. Radiother Oncol 2007;85:146–55.

12. Vauterin TJ, Veness MJ, Morgan GJ, et al. Patterns of lymph node spread of cutaneous squamous cell carcinoma of the head and neck. Head Neck 2006;28:785–91.

13. Wang Y, Ow TJ, Myers JN. Pathways for cervical metastasis in malignant neoplasms of the head and neck region. Clin Anat 2012;25:54–71.

14. Taylor BW Jr, Brant TA, Mendenhall NP, et al. Carcinoma of the skin metastatic to parotid area lymph nodes. Head Neck 1991;13:427–33.

15. Marks NJ. The anatomy of the lymph nodes of the parotid gland. Clin Otolaryngol Allied Sci 1984;9:271–5.

16. McKean ME, Lee K, McGregor IA. The distribution of lymph nodes in and around the parotid gland: an anatomical study. Br J Plast Surg 1985;38:1–5.

17. Carmeliet P, Jain RK. Angiogenesis in cancer and other diseases. Nature 2001;407:249–57.

18. Ji RC. Lymphatic endothelial cells, tumor lymphangiogenesis and metastasis: new insights into intratumoral and peritumoral lymphatics. Cancer Metastasis Rev 2006;25:677–94.

19. Karpanen T, Egeblad M, Karkkainen MJ, et al. Vascular endothelial growth factor C promotes tumor lymphangiogenesis and intralymphatic tumor growth. Cancer Res 2001;61:1786–90.

20. Jüttner S, Wissmann C, Jöns T, et al. Vascular endothelial growth factor-D and its receptor VEGFR-3: two novel independent prognostic markers in gastric adenocarcinoma. J Clin Oncol 2006;24:228–40.

21. Laakkonen P, Waltari M, Holopainen T, et al. Vascular endothelial growth factor receptor 3 is involved in tumor angiogenesis and growth. Cancer Res 2007; 67:593–9.

22. Sugiura T, Inoue Y, Matsuki R, et al. VEGF-C and VEGF-D expression is correlated with lymphatic vessel density and lymph node metastasis in oral squamous cell carcinoma: implications for use as a prognostic marker. Int J Oncol 2009; 34:673–80.

23. Bo C, Xiaopeng D, Chuanliang P, et al. Expression of vascular endothelial growth factors C and D correlates with lymphangiogenesis and lymph node metastasis in lung adenocarcinoma. Thorac Cardiovasc Surg 2009;57:291–4.

24. Achen MG, Stacker SA. Molecular control of lymphatic metastasis. Ann N Y Acad Sci 2008; 1131:225–34.

25. Nathanson SD. Insights into the mechanisms of lymph node metastasis. Cancer 2003;98:413–23.

26. Cho SB, Chung WG, Yun M, et al. Fluorodeoxyglucose positron emission tomography in cutaneous squamous cell carcinoma: retrospective analysis of 12 patients. Dermatol Surg 2005;31:442–6.

27. Knappe M, Louw M, Gregor RT. Ultrasonography-guided fine-needle aspiration for the assessment of cervical metastases. Arch Otolaryngol Head Neck Surg 2000;126:1091–6.

28. Ross AS, Schmults CD. Sentinel lymph node biopsy in cutaneous squamous cell carcinoma: a systematic review of the English literature. Dermatol Surg 2006; 32:1309–21.

29. Farasat S, Yu SS, Neel VA, et al. A new American Joint Committee on Cancer staging system for cutaneous squamous cell carcinoma: creation and rationale for inclusion of tumor (T) characteristics. J Am Acad Dermatol 2011;64:1051–9.

30. Breuninger H, Brantsch K, Eigentler T, et al. Comparison and evaluation of the current staging of cutaneous carcinomas. J Dtsch Dermatol Ges 2012; 10(8):579–86.

31. O'Brien CJ, McNeil EB, McMahon JD, et al. Significance of clinical stage, extent of surgery, and pathologic findings in metastatic cutaneous squamous carcinoma of the parotid gland. Head Neck 2002; 24:417–22.

32. Andruchow JL, Veness MJ, Morgan GJ, et al. Implications for clinical staging of metastatic cutaneous squamous carcinoma of the head and neck based on a multicenter study of treatment outcomes. Cancer 2006;106:1078–83.

33. Forest VI, Clark JJ, Veness MJ, et al. N1S3: a revised staging system for head and neck cutaneous squamous cell carcinoma with lymph node

metastases: results of 2 Australian Cancer Centers. Cancer 2010;116:1298–304.

34. Palme CE, MacKay SG, Kalnis I, et al. The need for a better prognostic staging system in patients with metastatic cutaneous squamous cell carcinoma of the head and neck. Curr Opin Otolaryngol Head Neck Surg 2007;15:103–6.

35. O'Hara J, Ferlito A, Takes RP, et al. Cutaneous squamous cell carcinoma of the head and neck metastasizing to the parotid gland—a review of current recommendations. Head Neck 2011;33:1789–95.

36. Iyer NG, Clark JR, Murali R, et al. Outcomes following parotidectomy for metastatic squamous cell carcinoma with microscopic residual disease: implications for facial nerve preservation. Head Neck 2009;31:21–7.

37. Veness MJ, Porceddu S, Palme CE, et al. Cutaneous head and neck squamous cell carcinoma metastatic to parotid and cervical lymph nodes. Head Neck 2007;29:621–31.

38. Dona E, Veness MJ, Cakir B, et al. Metastatic cutaneous squamous cell carcinoma to the parotid: the role of surgery and adjuvant radiotherapy to achieve best outcome. ANZ J Surg 2003;73:692–6.

39. Chen AM, Grekin RC, Garcia J, et al. Radiation therapy for cutaneous squamous cell carcinoma involving the parotid area lymph nodes: dose and volume considerations. Int J Radiat Oncol Biol Phys 2007;69:1377–80.

40. Mendenhall WM, Amdur RJ, Hinerman RW, et al. Radiotherapy for cutaneous squamous and basal cell carcinomas of the head and neck. Laryngoscope 2009;119:1994–9.

41. Audet N, Palme CE, Gullane PJ, et al. Cutaneous metastatic squamous cell carcinoma to the parotid gland: analysis and outcome. Head Neck 2004;26: 727–32.

42. Ying YM, Johnson JT, Myers EN. Squamous cell carcinoma of the parotid gland. Head Neck 2006; 28:626–32.

43. Moore BA, Weber RW, Prieto V, et al. Lymph node metastases from cutaneous squamous cell carcinoma of the head and neck. Laryngoscope 2005; 115:1561–7.

44. Kirke DN, Porceddu S, Wallwork BD, et al. Pathologic occult neck disease in patients with metastatic cutaneous squamous cell carcinoma to the parotid. Otolaryngol Head Neck Surg 2011;144: 549–51.

45. Ebrahimi A, Moncrieff MD, Clark JR, et al. Predicting the pattern of regional metastases from cutaneous squamous cell carcinoma of the head and neck based on location of the primary. Head Neck 2010; 32:1288–94.

46. Osborne RF, Shaw T, Zandifar H, et al. Elective parotidectomy in the management of advanced auricular malignancies. Laryngoscope 2008;118: 2139–45.

47. Yoon M, Chougule P, Dufresne R, et al. Localized carcinoma of the external ear is an unrecognized aggressive disease with a high propensity for local regional recurrence. Am J Surg 1992;164:574–7.

48. Peiffer N, Kutz JW Jr, Myers LL, et al. Patterns of regional metastasis in advanced stage cutaneous squamous cell carcinoma of the auricle. Otolaryngol Head Neck Surg 2011;144:36–42.

49. DeConti RC. Chemotherapy of squamous cell carcinoma of the skin. Semin Oncol 2012;39:145–9.

50. Wollina U. Cetuximab in non-melanoma skin cancer. Expert Opin Biol Ther 2012;12(7):949–56.

Uncommon Cutaneous Neoplasms of the Head and Neck

David R. Reinstadler, MD, Uttam K. Sinha, MD*

KEYWORDS

- Neoplasm • Skin cancer • Head and neck cancer • Cutaneous cancer

KEY POINTS

- In what was once a disease of older generations, the overall incidence of cutaneous malignancies continues to increase, with a disproportionate increase in younger patients likely as a result of increasing sun exposure.
- UVB rays cause most damage associated with carcinogenesis, as a consequence of energy absorption in different skin layers. UVA rays penetrate deeper into the dermis resulting in solar elastosis, whereas UVB rays are almost completely absorbed by the epidermis.
- Public education is the first step in curbing the increase in potentially preventable neoplasms.

INTRODUCTION

The lifetime risk for any American to develop some form of skin cancer has been estimated to be one in five.[1] A large proportion of these cutaneous malignancies fall into the category of nonmelanoma skin cancer with malignant melanoma comprising a smaller proportion. Incidence of nonmelanoma skin cancer has been reported to be 18 to 20 times greater than that of malignant melanoma.[2] Within the category of nonmelanoma skin cancer, the ratio of basal cell carcinoma to squamous cell carcinoma is approximately 4:1.[3] In what was formerly a disease of older generations, the overall incidence of these malignancies continues to increase, with a disproportionate increase in younger patients likely caused by increasing sun exposure.[4,5]

Ultraviolet (UV) radiation exposure is a significant inciting or contributing factor in almost all cutaneous malignancies. Within the UV spectrum, it has been shown that UVB rays (290–320 nm) cause most damage associated with carcinogenesis, whereas UVA rays (320–400 nm) contribute to overall age-related changes in the skin.[6] This is partly caused by the site of energy absorption in different skin layers. UVA rays penetrate deeper into the dermis resulting in solar elastosis, whereas UVB rays are almost completely absorbed by the epidermis.[7] The absorption of UVA radiation also is predominantly by non-DNA chromophores, leading to indirect DNA damage through the creation of reactive oxygen species causing single strand breaks.[8] This is less traumatic than UVB radiation causing direct DNA damage through dimer formation.[9] The primary process responsible for repair of damaged DNA is the nucleotide excision repair mechanism.[10] If this mechanism is overwhelmed, usually through continuous or repeated UV exposure, the damage goes unrepaired. When these mutations affect genes encoding regulatory functions, uncontrolled proliferation occurs. The most well-studied mutation is with the p53 tumor suppressor gene.[7]

Basal cell carcinoma and squamous cell carcinoma comprise most nonmelanoma skin cancers. Other histologic forms, such as Merkel cell

There are no conflicts of interest or financial disclosures to be made in this manuscript.
Department of Otolaryngology–Head and Neck Surgery, University of Southern California, 1200 North State Street, #4136, Los Angeles, CA 90033, USA
* Corresponding author.
E-mail address: sinha@med.usc.edu

facialplastic.theclinics.com

carcinoma (MCC), atypical fibroxanthoma (AFX), malignant fibrous histiocytoma (MFH), dermatofibrosarcoma protuberans (DFSP), microcystic adnexal carcinoma (MAC), and sebaceous carcinoma, are also described in this category, although their incidence is much lower. There is abundant information in the literature on basal cell carcinoma and squamous cell carcinoma. This article concentrates on the less-common malignancies.

MCC

MCC is a relatively new tumor, previously called trabecular carcinoma or cutaneous neuroendocrine carcinoma. The Merkel cell is the only cutaneous cell known to contain neurosecretory granules and resides in the basal layer of the epidermis. There is still debate as to whether the Merkel cell is of neuroendocrine origin[11] or a puripotent stem cell.[12] Even the function of these cells remains to be fully understood, although they are thought to play a role in mechanoreception and endocrine signaling.[13] They do, however, form a very small but aggressive portion of the nonmelanoma skin cancers.

The incidence of MCC in the United States is estimated to be between 0.32 and 0.44 per 100,000 person-years.[14,15] Males have a higher incidence than females at approximately 2:1, and whites have approximately eight times the risk of blacks.[14] MCC is rare in persons younger than age 50 years, then increases between ages 50 and 65.[14] Like other nonmelanoma skin cancers, the incidence increases in areas of higher UV exposure, with the most common location being on the head and neck (48%), upper limb (19%), lower limb (16%), and trunk (11%).[14]

The cause of MCC has not been completely elucidated. Many contributing factors are being suggested and trends have been observed, but no definitive factors have been reported. MCC has been seen in many forms of immunosuppression, both autoimmune and iatrogenic.[16–19] There have been reports of partial regression of metastatic lesions after discontinuation of immunosuppression.[20,21] This risk is not specific to MCC, because the risks of other malignancies also increase with any degree of immunosuppression.

UV radiation is strongly associated with the development of MCC. Although no conclusive evidence has shown causation, their occurrence within a background of solar elastosis, Actinic keratoses, and other UV-induced changes strongly suggests a contributing effect.[22] Mutations in the p53 tumor suppressor gene have also been identified in MCC,[23] a change considered diagnostic of UV-induced DNA damage.[24] Patients with psoriasis undergoing psoralen-UVA

therapy have shown a 100-fold increase over the general population in incidence of MCC, indicating UVA along with UVB radiation plays a role.

Viral infection has been the most studied and promising etiologic factor. Recently, Feng and colleagues[25] characterized a new polyomavirus, Merkel cell polyomavirus. Approximately 80% of individuals older than 50 years show seropositivity to Merkel cell polyomavirus,[26] although little is known about transmission and latency. Since this discovery, many groups have published data on prevalence of Merkel cell polyomavirus DNA in MCC lesions, with rates ranging from 40%[27] to 100%.[28] Further research is needed to determine the virus' role in carcinogenesis.

Commonly, MCC develops as an asymptomatic rapidly growing nodule (over 6–12 months).[29] The tumor is usually flesh colored, firm, and nontender. There may be overlying telangiectasia and the differential diagnosis may include a simple cyst, basal cell carcinoma, adnexal tumor, amelanotic melanoma, or other nondescript cutaneous lesion. Diagnosis is established by biopsy (**Fig. 1**).

Immunohistochemistry is important in the diagnosis, because the histopathology can be similar to other cutaneous malignancies. MCC is positive for epithelial (CK20) and neuroendocrine (NFP) markers, whereas lacking markers for lymphoid or melanoma lesions.[30]

Since its description, multiple staging systems have been discussed. Only recently, a single system has emerged and gained universal acceptance. This staging system was recently published by the American Joint Committee on Cancer in their 7th edition, 2010 version, and maintains the standard T1 to T4 categories (**Tables 1** and **2**).[31]

Recurrence rates have been reported from 25% to 30%, regional lymph node involvement in 52%

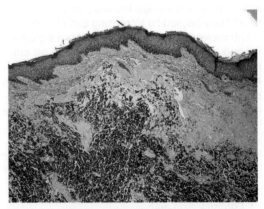

Fig. 1. Low-power view of Merkel cell carcinoma demonstrating a small round blue cell tumor forming nests or trabeculae.

Table 1
TNM criteria for Merkel cell carcinoma

T	N	M
Tx – primary tumor cannot be assessed	Nx – regional nodes cannot be assessed	Mx – distant metastasis cannot be assessed
T0 – no primary tumor	N0 – no regional node metastasis	M0 – no distant metastasis
Tis – in situ primary tumor	cN0 – nodes not clinically detectable	M1 – distant metastasis
T1 – primary tumor ≤2 cm	cN1 – nodes clinically detectable	M1a – distant skin, distant subcutaneous tissue, or distant lymph node metastasis
T2 – primary tumor ≥2 cm but ≤5 cm	pN0 – nodes negative by pathologic evaluation	M1b – lung metastasis
T3 – primary tumor >5 cm	pNx – nodes not evaluated pathologically	M1c – metastasis to all other visceral sites
T4 – primary tumor invades bone, muscle, fascia, or cartilage	N1a – micrometastasis N1b – macrometastasis N2 – in-transit metastasis	

Data from Lemos BD, Storer BE, Iyer JG, et al. Pathologic nodal evaluation improves prognostic accuracy in Merkel cell carcinoma: analysis of 5823 cases as the basis of the first consensus staging system. J Am Acad Dermatol 2010;63(5):751–61.

to 59%, and distant metastasis in 34% to 36% of all MCC.[32–34] This tumor carries a higher metastatic and mortality rate than malignant melanoma, so the treatment algorithm is much more aggressive.

Surgery is the primary treatment modality for MCC, although there is still debate on adjuvant therapy after resection. The current National Comprehensive Cancer Network guidelines[35] support the use of wide local excision with 1- to 2-cm margins or Mohs micrographic excision. Further treatment depends on involvement of primary lymph node drainage basins. Because of the high rate of lymph node involvement, sentinel lymph node biopsy is recommended.[36] Approximately one-third of patients are understaged if this is not done because of occult microscopic nodal involvement.[36] If sentinel lymph node biopsy is positive, completion neck dissection or radiation therapy is indicated. The use of radiation therapy after excision has been shown to improve local and regional recurrence rates.[37] Radiation therapy alone has demonstrated control rates in 75% of primary lesions.[38] Either primary or adjuvant chemotherapy has been used mainly for metastatic disease, but no survival benefit seems to be gained by its use.[39]

The overall 5-year survival of MCC is around 62%.[40] The 5-year survival rate for patients with local disease only is 64%, whereas survival for patients with nodal disease and distant metastasis decreases to 39% and 18%, respectively.[31] This low survival for local disease is largely caused by the discrepancy between T1 lesions (stage IA, 79% 5-year survival) and T4 lesions (stage IIC, 47% 5-year survival), which both fall into this category.[31] Primary lesions on the upper limb and younger age are independently associated with a better prognosis.[40]

A mucosal variant is also seen but at a much lower incidence. The most commonly affected site is the larynx, followed by nasal cavity, pharynx, and the mouth and tongue.[40] This has a much poorer prognosis than cutaneous MCC with the overall survival rate being 49% at 2 years.

Table 2
Merkel cell carcinoma staging

Stage	Stage Grouping		
0	Tis	N0	M0
IA	T1	pN0	M0
IB	T1	cN0	M0
IIA	T2/T3	pN0	M0
IIB	T2/T3	cN0	M0
IIC	T4	N0	M0
IIIA	Any T	N1a	M0
IIIB	Any T	N1b/N2	M0
IV	Any T	Any N	M1

Data from Lemos BD, Storer BE, Iyer JG, et al. Pathologic nodal evaluation improves prognostic accuracy in Merkel cell carcinoma: analysis of 5823 cases as the basis of the first consensus staging system. J Am Acad Dermatol 2010;63(5):751–61.

AFX AND MFH

AFX is a fibrohistiocytic tumor, 75% of which occur on the head and neck.[41] It was first described in 1961 as a dermal tumor exhibiting a benign course[42–44] and thought to arise from actinic and UV damage.[45] This lesion arises, like many other UV-induced tumors, in older white males (seventh decade) with a male/female ratio approaching 7:1.[41,46] Because of the rarity of this tumor, there are not specific incidence rates available.

Clinical presentation of AFX is commonly that of a single friable nodule less than 2 cm. Diagnosis is made with biopsy showing atypical spindle and polygonal cells arranged haphazardly (**Fig. 2**).[47] This histologic appearance may be indistinguishable from a more aggressive entity, MFH, which many believe to be a variation of the same tumor. Immunostains may be helpful in distinguishing this spindle cell lesion from other malignancies, such as spindle cell squamous cell carcinoma, although there is not a high degree of specificity for confirming the diagnosis itself.[48]

MFH occurs most commonly on the head and neck but also has a significant incidence on the extremities.[41] It usually occurs in a slightly younger age group, in the fifth to seventh decade. The presentation is usually more striking than that of AFX, with a 5- to 10-cm nodule or ulceration.[44] Because the cellular morphology is similar in AFX and MFH, the pathologist must use other features to make a distinction. Deep invasion into the subcutaneous tissue, necrosis, or perineural or perivascular invasion are findings that tip the diagnosis in favor of MFH.[41] Although similar in their immunohistochemical profile, MFH tends to show strong positivity for CD74 and negative staining for CD99.[49,50] AFX is only weakly positive for CD74 and positive for CD99 in 35% to 75% of cases.[50,51]

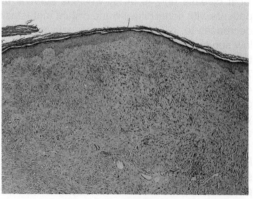

Fig. 2. Low-power view of atypical fibroxanthoma showing haphazardly arranged spindle-shaped cells.

Treatment of AFX is generally much less aggressive than MFH. Wide local excision and Mohs surgery are the favored modalities, although radiation and cryotherapy have been reported. The latter options are not preferred because of the inability to assess margins and possibility to increase the aggressive behavior.[52] The recurrence rate is around 10% for wide local excision and it is recommended to take 1- to 2-cm margins with the deep margin being to the fascial plane.[46,53] When using Mohs micrographic surgery, the recurrence rate is significantly reduced because of the subclinical extension outside normal excision margins.[46] There have been reported cases of metastatic AFX, although many authors believe these were incorrectly classified and likely represented MFH versus spindle cell squamous cell carcinoma.[54]

Management of MFH consists of resection either with wide local excision or Mohs micrographic surgery. Wide local excision has shown recurrence rates up to 71% likely caused by the highly infiltrative growth pattern.[55] No specific parameters have been set on the margins required for clearance, but it is accepted to use at least 2 cm around clinically apparent tumor. Magnetic resonance imaging or other imaging modalities have been recommended in cases of deeply penetrating tumors. Deep margins should include fascia, soft tissue, or bone, dictated by tumor extent. Metastasis has been reported in up to 44% of cases, although this number is reduced to 18% when the tumor is limited to subcuticular tissue.[56,57] Tumor size and histologic grade seem to have the greatest impact on survival. Tumors less than 5 cm have a 79% 5-year survival, whereas when lesions are between 5 and 10 cm and more than 10 cm, survival rates drop to 63% and 41%, respectively.[57]

DFSP

DFSP is a rare soft tissue malignancy occurring most often on the trunk and less commonly in the head and neck. The annual incidence is approximately 4.2 to 4.5 per million.[58,59] Unlike other cutaneous malignancies, persons age 24 to 50 years have the highest likelihood of developing this tumor,[60] with 80% occurring in this group. Overall local recurrence rates have been reported as high as 60%[60] although the rate of distant metastasis is extremely low.

This lesion most commonly presents as a painless subcutaneous nodule and can be mistaken for scar tissue on physical examination, growing slowly over years. Plaque-like lesions of varying color may also be observed. Microscopically, a dense network of monomorphic fusiform cells forming cartwheel configurations is seen. Mitoses are rare, congruent with its low-grade behavior. Many deep, finger-like projections are present, making borders indistinct and accounting for high recurrence rates. Immunohistochemistry is useful in discriminating between DFSP and dermatofibroma, with DFSP avidly staining positive for CD34 and negative for factor XIIIa (**Fig. 3**).[61] DFSP have been characterized by a specific chromosomal translocation, t(17;22)(q22;q13),[62] with this demonstrated in more than 90% of lesions. This translocation leads to overexpression of platelet-derived growth factor receptor β.[63]

The treatment of choice is surgical removal either with traditional wide local excision or Mohs technique. With the use of wide local excision, 2- to 4-cm margins are needed, with deep margins extending to the underlying investing fascia.[64] A recent review compared recurrence rates between wide excision and Mohs and found no statically significant difference.[65] Radiation therapy has been used, mostly as an adjuvant to excision, but also in cases of unresectable tumors. Newer therapies are being investigated, including imatinib mesylate, a tyrosine kinase inhibitor active against tumors displaying the chromosomal translocation.[66] It has recently gained approval from the Food and Drug Administration for treatment of unresectable, recurrent, or metastatic lesions.[67]

MAC

MAC is another rare cutaneous tumor with only around 300 cases reported in the literature.[68] The most common primary site is the head and neck (88%), with most occurring on the central face (73%).[69] White patients represent most of the cases with fewer than 10 cases described in blacks.[70] UV and ionizing radiation, along with immunosuppression, are thought to be risk factors, although no definitive association has been made.[71]

Clinical presentation varies, but most present as flesh-colored, smooth, asymptomatic nodules, the growth pattern of which seems to be indolent. Microscopically, the tumor infiltrates the reticular and papillary dermis, sparing the epidermis and displaying small cysts with keratinization.[72] In some areas there are interspersed basal cells forming ducts with well-defined lumens.[73] The clinical and histopathologic diagnosis can be difficult, and many cases are misdiagnosed as basal cell carcinoma (**Fig. 4**).[74]

Although this tumor rarely metastasizes, recurrence rates up to 60% make this tumor difficult to treat.[74] It has a propensity for perineural invasion, with recurrent tumors displaying this feature in 87.5% of cases.[75] Extensive subclinical extension into the subcutaneous tissue and adjacent normal-looking tissue also contribute to the difficulty in complete excision. The high recurrence rates are usually caused by the fact that there are no accepted safe margins for conventional excision because of its infiltrative pattern. For this reason, Mohs has been suggested as the treatment of choice,[68] with recurrence rates ranging from 0% to 12%.[69,76]

SEBACEOUS CARCINOMA

Sebaceous carcinoma is a rare malignancy of the adnexal structures of the dermis and subcutaneous tissue. It occurs most commonly on the head and neck and has a propensity for occurring on the eyelid in association with the meibomian glands.[77,78] A recent review of the Surveillance, epidemiology, and end results (SEER) database[78] evaluated 1836 cases of sebaceous carcinoma and found a slight male predominance (55%) occurring at an average age of 70. Forty-two percent of the tumors occurred on the face, ear, scalp, neck, and lip, with 34% occurring on the eyelid. Therefore, this tumor is normally classified

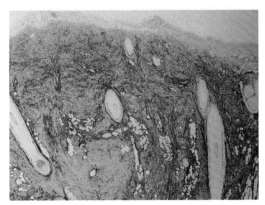

Fig. 3. Immunohistochemistry of dermatofibrosarcoma protuberans staining avidly for CD34.

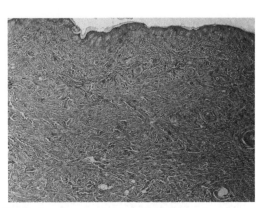

Fig. 4. Low-power view of microcystic adnexal carcinoma demonstrating superficial keratocysts infiltrating the dermis and sparing the epidermis.

by location as ocular or extraocular. The underlying cause is not well understood, although these lesions tend not to occur from pre-existing sebaceous conditions.[79]

A varied clinical presentation makes the initial diagnosis of this tumor difficult. Extraocular lesions commonly present as a firm papule with a yellow hue because of the high fat content. Ocular lesions tend to mimic a common chalazion and diagnosis may be delayed. Ocular lesions may also present as diffuse lid erythema and edema resembling multiple more common inflammatory processes. Biopsy is essential for the correct diagnosis. Histologic evaluation shows aggregates of neoplastic cells centered in the deep dermis.[80] Intraepithelial spread of neoplastic cells is the classic identifier for this tumor[47] along with many specimens showing abundant lipid content when properly stained (**Fig. 5**).[81] Extraocular tumors are less likely to exhibit intraepithelial spread.[47] Immunohistochemical stains may be helpful in some cases of ambiguous histology. Sebaceous carcinoma stains positive for epithelial membrane antigen and androgen receptors, but is negative for carcinoembryonic antigen and S100.[81]

Muir-Torre syndrome is important to evaluate for when a diagnosis of sebaceous carcinoma is confirmed. This autosomal-dominant genodermatosis has mutations in MLH1 and MSH2, which are involved in DNA mismatch repair. Clinically, this syndrome consists of one sebaceous neoplasm of the skin and one low-grade visceral malignancy, most commonly colorectal and genitourinary.[81] Further work-up is necessary when a diagnosis of Muir-Torre syndrome is suspected.

Excision is the mainstay of treatment for this tumor. Because of the infiltrative nature of the ocular lesions, Mohs micrographic surgery is recommended.[82] Wide local excision may be used for the extraocular lesions; for more advanced lesions orbital exenteration may be necessary. Recurrence rates have been reported between 6% and 36% at 5 years.[81,83] Regional lymph node metastasis is reported at 2.4%.[78] Ocular tumors have an overall higher rate of lymph node involvement (4.4%) compared with the extraocular location (1.4%).[78] Poorly differentiated tumors metastasized to lymph nodes at a rate of 13.9%, whereas well-differentiated tumors showed no metastasis according to the recent SEER database review.[78] With this information, sentinel lymph node biopsy is recommended for poorly differentiated and ocular lesions.[78,84]

SUMMARY

With the incidence of nonmelanoma skin cancers continuing to rise, knowledge of these conditions is necessary for all clinicians. New research into the cause and genetics of these malignancies provides avenues for further diagnostic and treatment strategies. With most of these malignancies arising from sun-damaged skin, prevention and regular skin screenings are paramount. Public education is the first step in curbing the increase in these potentially preventable neoplasms.

ACKNOWLEDGMENTS

The authors thank the Department of Dermatology at the University of California Irvine for histology photos.

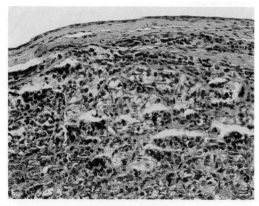

Fig. 5. Sebaceous carcinoma showing multiple foamy cells with vacuolated cytoplasm.

REFERENCES

1. Rigel DS, Friedman RJ, Kopf AW. Lifetime risk for development of skin cancer in the US population: current estimate is now 1 in 5. J Am Acad Dermatol 1996;35(6):1012–3.
2. Diepgen TL, Mahler V. The epidemiology of skin cancer. Br J Dermatol 2002;146(Suppl 61):1–6.
3. Silverberg E, Boring CC, Squires TS. Cancer statistics 1990. CA Cancer J Clin 1990;40:9–26.
4. Christenson LJ, Borrowman TA, Vachon CM, et al. Incidence of basal cell and squamous cell carcinomas in a population younger than 40 years. JAMA 2005;294(6):681–90.
5. Hausauer AK, Swetter SM, Cockburn MG, et al. Increases in melanoma among adolescent girls and young women in California: trends by socioeconomic status and UV radiation exposure. Arch Dermatol 2011;147(7):783–9.
6. Berking C, Takemoto R, Binder RL, et al. Photocarcinogenesis in human adult skin grafts. Carcinogenesis 2002;23:181–7.

7. Rass K, Reichrath J. UV damage and DNA repair in malignant melanoma and nonmelanoma skin cancer. Adv Exp Med Biol 2008;624:162–78.

8. Peak JG, Peak MJ. Comparison of initial yields of DNA-to-protein crosslinks and single-strand breaks induced in cultured human cells by far- and near-ultraviolet light, blue light and X-rays. Mutat Res 1991;246:187–91.

9. Varghese AJ, Patrick MH. Cytosine derived het-croadduct formation in ultraviolet-irradiated DNA. Nature 1969;223:299–300.

10. Setlow RB, Carrier WL. The disappearance of thymine dimers from DNA: an error-correcting mechanism. Proc Natl Acad Sci U S A 1964;51:226–31.

11. Halata Z, Grim M, Bauman KI. Friedrich Sigmund Merkel and his "Merkel cell", morphology, development, and physiology: review and new results. Anat Rec A Discov Mol Cell Evol Biol 2003;271:225–39.

12. Hewitt JB, Sherif A, Kerr KM, et al. Merkel cell and squamous cell carcinomas arising in erythema ab igne. Br J Dermatol 1993;128:591–2.

13. Lucarz A, Brand G. Current considerations about Merkel cells. Eur J Cell Biol 2007;86(5):243–51 [Epub 2007 Mar 6].

14. Agelli M, Clegg LX. Epidemiology of primary Merkel cell carcinoma in the United States. J Am Acad Dermatol 2003;49(5):832–41.

15. Hodgson NC. Merkel cell carcinoma: changing incidence trends. J Surg Oncol 2005;89:1–4.

16. Gooptu C, Woollons A, Ross J, et al. Merkel cell carcinoma arising after therapeutic immunosuppression. Br J Dermatol 1997;137:637–41.

17. Nemoto I, Sato-Matsumura KC, Fujita Y, et al. Leukaemic dissemination of Merkel cell carcinoma in a patient with systemic lupus erythematosus. Clin Exp Dermatol 2008;33:270–2.

18. McLoone NM, McKenna K, Edgar D, et al. Merkel cell carcinoma in a patient with chronic sarcoidosis. Clin Exp Dermatol 2005;30:580–2.

19. Gianfreda M, Caiffi S, De Franceschi T, et al. Merkel cell carcinoma of the skin in a patient with myasthenia gravis. Minerva Med 2002;93:219–22.

20. Friedlaender MM, Rubinger D, Rosenbaum E, et al. Temporary regression of Merkel cell carcinoma metastases after cessation of cyclosporine. Transplantation 2002;73:1849–50.

21. Muirhead R, Ritchie DM. Partial regression of Merkel cell carcinoma in response to withdrawal of azathioprine in an immunosuppression-induced case of metastatic Merkel cell carcinoma. Clin Oncol (R Coll Radiol) 2007;19:96.

22. Aydin A, Kocer NE, Bekerecioglu M, et al. Cutaneous undifferentiated small (Merkel) cell carcinoma, that developed synchronously with multiple actinic keratoses, squamous cell carcinomas and basal cell carcinoma. J Dermatol 2003;30:241–4.

23. Popp S, Waltering S, Herbst C, et al. UV–B-type mutations and chromosomal imbalances indicate common pathways for the development of Merkel and skin squamous cell carcinomas. Int J Cancer 2002;99:352–60.

24. Ziegler A, Jonason AS, Leffell DJ, et al. Sunburn and p53 in the onset of skin cancer. Nature 1994;372:773–6.

25. Feng H, Shuda M, Chang Y, et al. Clonal integration of a polyomavirus in human Merkel cell carcinoma. Science 2008;319:1096–100.

26. Tolstov YL, Pastrana DV, Feng H, et al. Human Merkel cell polyomavirus infection II. MCV is a common human infection that can be detected by conformational capsid epitope immunoassays. Int J Cancer 2009;125:1250–6.

27. Wetzels CT, Hoefnagel JG, Bakkers JM, et al. Ultrastructural proof of polyomavirus in Merkel cell carcinoma tumour cells and its absence in small cell carcinoma of the lung. PLoS One 2009;4:e4958.

28. Sastre-Garau X, Peter M, Avril MF, et al. Merkel cell carcinoma of the skin: pathological and molecular evidence for a causative role of MCV in oncogenesis. J Pathol 2009;218:48–56.

29. Dancey AL, Rayatt SS, Soon C, et al. Merkel cell carcinoma: a report of 34 cases and literature review. J Plast Reconstr Aesthet Surg 2006;59:1294–9.

30. McCardle TW, Sondak VK, Zager J, et al. Merkel cell carcinoma: pathologic findings and prognostic factors. Curr Probl Cancer 2010;34:47–64.

31. Lemos BD, Storer BE, Iyer JG, et al. Pathologic nodal evaluation improves prognostic accuracy in Merkel cell carcinoma: analysis of 5823 cases as the basis of the first consensus staging system. J Am Acad Dermatol 2010;63(5):751–61.

32. Akhtar S, Oza KK, Wright J. Merkel cell carcinoma: report of 10 cases and review of the literature [review]. J Am Acad Dermatol 2000;43(5 Pt 1):755–67.

33. Medina-Franco H, Urist MM, Fiveash J, et al. Multimodality treatment of Merkel cell carcinoma: case series and literature review of 1024 cases. Ann Surg Oncol 2001;8(3):204–8.

34. Gillenwater AM, Hessel AC, Morrison WH, et al. Merkel cell carcinoma of the head and neck: effect of surgical excision and radiation on recurrence and survival. Arch Otolaryngol Head Neck Surg 2001;127(2):149–54.

35. Cited with permission from the NCCN Clinical Practice Guidelines in Oncology (NCCN Guidelines) for Merkel Cell Carcinoma V1.2011 © 2010 National Comprehensive Cancer Network, Inc. All rights reserved. The NCCN Guidelines and illustrations herein may not be reproduced in any form for any purpose without the express written permission of the NCCN. To view the most recent and complete version of the NCCN Guidelines, go online to NCCN.org. NATIONAL COMPREHENSIVE CANCER NETWORK, NCCN, NCCN GUIDELINES, and all

other NCCN Content are trademarks owned by the National Comprehensive Cancer Network, Inc.

36. Gupta SG, Wang LC, Peñas PF, et al. Sentinel lymph node biopsy for evaluation and treatment of patients with Merkel cell carcinoma: the Dana-Farber experience and meta-analysis of the literature. Arch Dermatol 2006;142(6):685–90.

37. Lewis KG, Weinstock MA, Weaver AL, et al. Adjuvant local irradiation for Merkel cell carcinoma. Arch Dermatol 2006;142(6):693–700.

38. Veness M, Foote M, Gebski V, et al. The role of radiotherapy alone in patients with Merkel cell carcinoma: reporting the Australian experience of 43 patients. Int J Radiat Oncol Biol Phys 2010;78(3):703–9 [Epub 2009 Nov 24].

39. Garneski KM, Nghiem P. Merkel cell carcinoma adjuvant therapy: current data support radiation but not chemotherapy. J Am Acad Dermatol 2007;57(1):166–9 [Epub 2007 May 7].

40. Agelli M, Clegg LX, Becker JC, et al. The etiology and epidemiology of Merkel cell carcinoma. Curr Probl Cancer 2010;34(1):14–37.

41. Withers A, Brougham N, Barber R, et al. Atypical fibroxanthoma and malignant fibrous histiocytoma. J Plast Reconstr Aesthet Surg 2011;64:e273–8.

42. Levan NE, Hirsch P, Kwong MQ. Pseudosarcomatous dermatofibroma. Arch Dermatol 1963;88:908–12.

43. Helwig EB. Atypical fibroxanthoma. Tex Med 1963;59:664–7.

44. Stadler FJ, Scott AS, Brown DB. Malignant fibrous tumours. Semin Cutan Med Surg 1998;17(2):141e52.

45. Dei Tos AP, Maestro R, Doglioni C, et al. Ultraviolet-induced p53 mutations in atypical fibroxanthoma. Am J Pathol 1994;145(1):11e7.

46. Davis JL, Randle HW, Zalla MJ, et al. A comparison of Mohs micrographic surgery and wide excision for the treatment of atypical fibroxanthoma. Dermatol Surg 1997;23:105–10.

47. Love W, Schmitt A, Bordeaux J. Cutaneous malignancies: atypical fibroxanthoma, malignant fibrous histiocytoma, sebaceous carcinoma, extramammary Paget disease. Dermatol Clin 2011;29:201–16.

48. Ma CK, Zarbo RJ, Gown AM. Immunohistochemical characterization of atypical fibroxanthoma and dermatofibrosarcoma protuberans. Am J Clin Pathol 1992;97:478–83.

49. Fletcher CD. Tumours of the skin. Diagnostic histopathology of tumours, vol. 23. 3rd edition. Philadelphia (PA): Elseiver Health Sciences; 2007. p. 1491–3.

50. Weedon D, Williamson R, Mirza B. CD10, a useful marker for atypical fibroxanthomas. Am J Dermatopathol 2005;27(2):181.

51. Hartel PH, Jackson J, Ducatman BS, et al. CD99 immunoreactivity in atypical fibroxanthoma and pleomorphic malignant fibrous histiocytoma: a useful diagnostic marker. J Cutan Pathol 2006;33(Suppl 2):24e8.

52. Jacoby WD Jr. Cryosurgical treatment of recurrent atypical fibroxanthoma of the skin. Preliminary report. Cutis 1978;22:599–601.

53. Starink TM, Hausman R, Van Delden L, et al. Atypical fibroxanthoma of the skin: presentation of 5 cases and review of the literature. Br J Dermatol 1977;97:167e77.

54. Brown MD. Atypical fibroxanthoma and malignant fibrous xanthoma. Surg Dermatol Adv Curr Pract. London (UK): Martin Dunitz publishing; 1993;1:201–10.

55. Kearney MM, Soule EH, Ivins JC. Malignant fibrous histiocytoma: a retrospective study of 167 cases. Cancer 1980;45:167–78.

56. Weiss SW, Enzinger FM. Malignant fibrous histiocytoma: an analysis of 200 cases. Cancer 1978;41:2250–66.

57. Pezzi CM, Rawlings MS Jr, Esgro JJ, et al. Prognostic factors in 227 patients with malignant fibrous histiocytoma. Cancer 1992;69:2098–103.

58. Criscione VD, Weinstock MA. Descriptive epidemiology of dermatofibrosarcoma protuberans in the United States, 1973 to 2002. J Am Acad Dermatol 2007;56(6):968–73 [Epub 2006 Dec 1].

59. Rouhani P, Fletcher CD, Devesa SS, et al. Cutaneous soft tissue sarcoma incidence patterns in the U.S.: an analysis of 12,114 cases. Cancer 2008;113(3):616–27.

60. Stojadinovic A, Karpoff HM, Antonescu CR, et al. Dermatofibrosarcoma protuberans of the head and neck. Ann Surg Oncol 2000;7(9):696–704.

61. Prieto VG, Reed JA, Shea CR. CD34 immunoreactivity distinguishes between scar tissue and residual tumor in re-excisional specimens of dermatofibrosarcoma protuberans. J Cutan Pathol 1994;21(4):324–9.

62. McArthur G. Dermatofibrosarcoma protuberans: recent clinical progress. Ann Surg Oncol 2007;14(10):2876–86.

63. Mendenhall WM, Zlotecki RA, Scarborough MT. Dermatofibrosarcoma protuberans [review]. Cancer 2004;101(11):2503–8.

64. Cited with permission from the NCCN Clinical Practice Guidelines in Oncology (NCCN Guidelines) for Dermatofibrosarcoma Protuberans V1.2011 © 2010 National Comprehensive Cancer Network, Inc. All rights reserved. The NCCN Guidelines and illustrations herein may not be reproduced in any form for any purpose without the express written permission of the NCCN. To view the most recent and complete version of the NCCN Guidelines, go online to NCCN.org. NATIONAL COMPREHENSIVE CANCER NETWORK, NCCN, NCCN GUIDELINES, and all other NCCN Content are trademarks owned by the National Comprehensive Cancer Network, Inc.

65. Meguerditchian AN, Wang J, Lema B, et al. Wide excision or Mohs micrographic surgery for the treatment of primary dermatofibrosarcoma protuberans. Am J Clin Oncol 2010;33(3):300–3.

66. Rubin BP, Schuetze SM, Eary JF, et al. Molecular targeting of platelet-derived growth factor B by imatinib mesylate in a patient with metastatic dermatofibrosarcoma protuberans. J Clin Oncol 2002;20(17): 3586–91.

67. McArthur GA. Molecular targeting of dermatofibrosarcoma protuberans: a new approach to a surgical disease. J Natl Compr Canc Netw 2007;5(5):557–62.

68. Wetter R, Goldstein GD. Microcystic adnexal carcinoma: a diagnostic and therapeutic challenge [review]. Dermatol Ther 2008;21(6):452–8.

69. Friedman P, Friedman R, Jiang B, et al. Microcystic adnexal carcinoma: collaborative series review and update. J Am Acad Dermatol 1999;41:225–31.

70. Nadiminti H, Nadiminti U, Washington C. Microcystic adnexal carcinoma in African-Americans. Dermatol Surg 2007;33:1384–7.

71. Cooper PH, Mills SE, Leonard DD, et al. Sclerosing sweat duct (syringomatous) carcinoma. Am J Surg Pathol 1985;9:422–33.

72. Martorell-Calatayud A, Requena-Caballero C, Botella-Estrada R, et al. Microcystic adnexal carcinoma: Mohs micrographic surgery as the treatment of choice. Actas Dermosifiliogr 2009;100:693–9.

73. Pujol RM, LeBoit PE, Su WP. Microcystic adnexal carcinoma with extensive sebaceous differentiation. Am J Dermatopathol 1997;19:358–62.

74. Chiller K, Passaro D, Scheuller M, et al. Microcystic adnexal carcinoma: forty-eight cases, their treatment, and their outcome. Arch Dermatol 2000;136: 1355–9.

75. Sebastien TS, Nelson BR, Lowe L. Microcystic adnexal carcinoma. J Am Acad Dermatol 1993;29:840–5.

76. Snow S, Madjar DD, Hardy S, et al. Microcystic adnexal carcinoma: report of 13 cases and review of the literature. Dermatol Surg 2001;27(4):401–8.

77. Rutten A, Wick MR, Sangueza O, et al. Sebaceous carcinoma. In: LeBoit P, Burg G, Weedon D, et al, editors. World Health Organization classification of tumors, pathology and genetics: skin tumors. Lyon (France): IARC Press; 2006. p. 160–3.

78. Tryggvason G, Bayon R, Pagedar NA. Epidemiology of sebaceous carcinoma of the head and neck: implications for lymph node management. Head Neck 2012. http://dx.doi.org/10.1002/hed.22009. [Epub ahead of print].

79. Shields JA, Demirci H, Marr BP, et al. Sebaceous carcinoma of the ocular region: a review. Surv Ophthalmol 2005;50:103–22.

80. Nelson BR, Hamlet KR, Gillard M, et al. Sebaceous carcinoma. J Am Acad Dermatol 1995;33:1–15.

81. Martinelli PT, Cohen PR, Schulze KE, et al. Sebaceous carcinoma. In: Nouri K, editor. Skin cancer. New York: McGraw-Hill; 2008. p. 240–50.

82. Thomas CJ, Wood GC, Marks VJ. Mohs micrographic surgery in the treatment of rare aggressive cutaneous tumors: the Geisinger experience. Dermatol Surg 2007;33:333–9.

83. Spencer JM, Nossa R, Tse DT, et al. Sebaceous carcinoma of the eyelid treated with Mohs micrographic surgery. J Am Acad Dermatol 2001;44: 1004–9.

84. Nijhawan N, Marriott C, Harvey JT. Lymphatic drainage patterns of the human eyelid: assessed by lymphoscintigraphy. Ophthal Plast Reconstr Surg 2010;26:281–5.

Nonmelanoma Skin Cancer of the Head and Neck: Reconstruction

Görkem Eskiizmir, MD[a], Shan Baker, MD[b],
Cemal Cingi, MD[c],*

KEYWORDS

- Reconstructive surgery • Skin cancer • Cutaneous cancer • Facial defects • Surgical technique

KEY POINTS

- A total excision of nonmelanoma skin cancer is a *sine qua non* for a successful reconstruction.
- Facial reconstruction should be tailored individually according to the defect, patient, and surgeon related factors.
- An accurate defect analysis and preoperative surgical plan should be performed and discussed with the patient.
- The major principles of facial reconstruction are helpful for obtaining the best surgical outcome.
- There is a learning curve in facial reconstruction that improves with surgical experience.

The face is the mirror of the soul.
—Cicero, a Roman philosopher (106 BC-43 BC)
De Oratore III, 22.

Beauty is the summation of the parts working together in such a way that nothing needed to be added, taken away or altered.
—Elio Carletti, an Italian impressionist artist (1925–1980).

INTRODUCTION

The face is a unique and complex feature that has functional and aesthetic importance. It is a source of social communication with emotions and expressions and provides vision, hearing, taste, smell, and even identity. Moreover, facial appearance may play a significant role in social life and relationships. Therefore, facial disfigurements or irregularities after skin cancer excision may lead to psychologic and social problems.

Facial reconstructive surgery aims to reestablish a "normal" face as closely as possible. In anatomic and aesthetic sense, a face is mainly divided into central and peripheral units. Both of these units topographically involve several facial aesthetic units and subunits that are constituted according to skin quality, thickness, color, texture, and contour. The central unit involves nose, lip, and eyelid; the peripheral unit involves cheek and forehead. Reconstruction of every facial unit is a challenge and should be tailored according to the following factors: defect related (size, shape, location, and thickness); patient related (comorbidities, habits expectancies, and so forth); surgeon related (experience).

A facial defect has three-dimensional topography. Therefore, the size, shape, and thickness of the defect should be evaluated precisely. In addition, the most effective surgical technique should be determined according to the location of the defect, and the adjacent skin elasticity should be examined, especially if a flap is required.

A candidate for facial reconstructive surgery should be evaluated in a physical and psychologic manner. The patient should be examined for comorbidities, such as diabetes mellitus, cardiovascular pathologies, and hypertension, which may cause a potential risk of complications. In addition,

[a] Department of Otolaryngology, Faculty of Medicine, Celal Bayar University, Manisa, Turkey; [b] Facial Plastic and Reconstructive Surgery, Department of Otolaryngology Head and Neck Surgery, University of Michigan, MI, USA; [c] Department of Otorhinolaryngology, Faculty of Medicine, Eskisehir Osmangazi University, Eskisehir, Turkey
* Corresponding author.
E-mail address: ccingi@gmail.com

Facial Plast Surg Clin N Am 20 (2012) 493–513
http://dx.doi.org/10.1016/j.fsc.2012.08.003
1064-7406/12/$ – see front matter © 2012 Elsevier Inc. All rights reserved.

the smoking status of a patient should be reviewed preoperatively, because the risk of graft or flap necrosis significantly increases in active smokers. Therefore, surgeons should encourage the patient to quit smoking at least 2 to 3 weeks before surgery. In addition, a delayed flap may be a better surgical option for active smokers. Finally, the functional and aesthetic outcomes and potential complications of surgery should be explained and discussed with the patient objectively.

This article focuses on the major surgical techniques used for the reconstruction of different facial units after nonmelanoma skin cancer excision.

RECONSTRUCTION OF THE NOSE

The nose is a masterpiece because of its anatomy, physiology, and aesthetic appearance. It is aesthetically subdivided into five subunits according to natural creases or boundaries: (1) dorsum, (2) sidewalls, (3) alar regions, (4) tip, and (5) columella. The topography (convexity or concavity), skin thickness, and texture are distinctive in each subunit. Depending on these differences, Burget and Menick suggested the "subunit" principle, which involves the excision of remaining healthy skin and reconstruction of an entire nasal subunit, when the defect involved 50% or greater surface area of the subunit.[1,2] They emphasized that this principle is helpful to camouflage incisions lines and creates inconspicuous scars, thereby providing aesthetically better outcomes. In contrast, Rohrich and coworkers[3] recommend preservation of all healthy skin and reconstruction of only the defect area, not the subunit.

The nose consist of three layers: (1) outer covering (skin, subcutaneous tissue, and muscles); (2) framework (nasal bones, quadrangular cartilage, upper and lower lateral cartilages); and (3) inner lining (mucoperichondrium/periosteum and skin of the nasal vestibule). The loss of each layer should be reconstructed individually and the ideal surgical technique of nasal reconstruction should be selected according to the size, shape, thickness, and location of the defect (**Fig. 1**).[4]

In nasal reconstruction, primary closure is the easiest surgical technique and, when possible, provides the best aesthetic outcome. It can be successfully applied to small (<1.5 cm in size) nasal defects that are located on the dorsum or sidewalls. Unfortunately, primary closure may lead to alar notching and tip deformities when used to repair moderate (1.5–2.5 cm in size) and large (>2.5 cm in size) defects of alar region and nasal tip.

Healing by secondary intention is rarely preferred for the aesthetic reconstruction of the nose. However, Zitelli emphasized that healing by secondary intention may offer an acceptable aesthetic outcome to patients who have nasal defects located on the concave surfaces of the nose.[5,6] Recently, an objective study supported this assumption and showed that small and superficial nasal defects that are located at the medial canthus can heal with an excellent aesthetic outcome.[7]

Full-thickness skin grafts can be technically performed to repair any defect that involves the outer covering of the nose, although they are best suited for dorsum, sidewall, and infratip region. However,

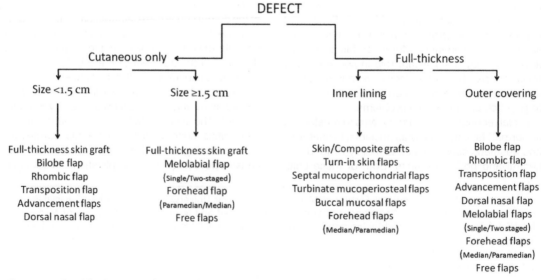

Fig. 1. An algorithmic approach to nasal reconstruction.

the aesthetic outcome of skin grafting in nasal reconstruction is generally less than expected. In a retrospective study, the clinical outcome of skin grafting and using skin flaps on the nose were examined and compared subjectively and objectively.[8] The authors demonstrated that texture mismatch and hypopigmentation are more likely after skin grafting. Therefore, postoperative skin resurfacing is generally offered to minimize the "patchy" appearance resulting in a better aesthetic outcome.[9]

Local Flaps

Local nasal flaps are technically formed by using the healthy remaining skin tissue of the nose. The most commonly used local nasal flaps are[10,11]:

- Bilobed flap
- Rhombic flap
- Advancement flap (Rintala flap)
- Dorsal nasal flap (Rieger flap)
- Transposition flap (note flap)

The most important advantage of local nasal flaps is in providing the ideal skin color, thickness, and texture match for the defect area. An excellent aesthetic outcome can be achieved if the most suitable flap design is selected.

The bilobed flap is generally preferred for small defects, especially if located on the caudal part of dorsum, supratip, tip, and alar regions. Rhombic flap can be especially helpful for rhombus-shaped small and moderate defects of dorsum or sidewall. Rintala flap is a one-stage flap harvested by advancement of skin of the nasal dorsum and glabellar region and mainly used for the reconstruction of small-to-moderate defects that are located on the dorsum and supratip region.[12]

The dorsal nasal flap, also called Rieger flap, is supplied by the angular artery and harvested by the rotation and partial advancement of nasal dorsal and glabella skin. It is an ideal surgical technique for the reconstruction of small-to-moderate defects of the middle and distal third of the nose.[13] Although local nasal flaps are generally used for the reconstruction of the outer covering of the nose, Wentzell[14] advocated that this technique can be successfully performed for the reconstruction of full-thickness nasal defects without using structural grafting and inner lining.

Local nasal flaps depend on the amount of remaining skin tissue, which is generally inadequate in large nasal defects; therefore, regional flaps should be considered when considerable skin is required for nasal reconstruction. In addition, the reliability of local flaps for the reconstruction of full-thickness nasal defects is low, because their blood supply is mostly based on a subcutaneous and intradermal vascular plexus (except dorsal nasal flap). Therefore, local nasal flaps may not adequately nourish cartilage grafts used for the nasal framework.

Regional Flaps

Regional flaps are the workhorse for reconstruction of large or full-thickness nasal defects. They are designed to recruit skin from adjacent areas, such as cheek and forehead. The skin laxity of these donor areas provides much more redundant skin to construct a flap compared with the nasal skin. The most frequently used regional flaps are:

- Rotation flap: classic glabellar flap
- Advancement flap: VY advancement cheek flap
- Transposition flaps: finger flap, single-stage melolabial flap
- Interpolated flaps: two-stage melolabial flap, paramedian/median forehead flap

The classic glabellar flap offers adequate redundant skin for the reconstruction of the upper one-third of the nose including medial canthus. Also, a finger flap can be designed in the glabella area and can be used for similar defects. Jackson[12] emphasized the finger flap as the most versatile surgical technique for the reconstruction of defects that are located in the medial canthus. VY advancement cheek flaps are technically easy to execute and a good surgical technique for the reconstruction of small-to-moderate defects of nasal sidewall. However, it may lead to loss of the nasofacial sulcus and a second surgery may be required to restore the sulcus. Melolabial flaps, either single- or two-stage, are ideally suited for the reconstruction of the alar region and sidewall by having an excellent match in skin color and texture with the adjacent nasal skin and exhibitins minimal donor site scarring.

Melolabial Flap

Thornton and Weathers[15] emphasized that an aesthetically satisfactory outcome can be obtained when melolabial flaps are performed to repair properly selected nasal tip defects. A single-stage melolabial flap is a transposition flap. The most important drawback of single-stage melolabial flap is the potential risk of trap-door deformity and distortion or loss of alar-facial sulcus, thereby causing an unsatisfactory aesthetic outcome. Nevertheless, Fazio and Zitelli[16] described a modified single-stage melolabial flap and stated that this technique provides excellent outcome with minimal risk of complication. In contrast, Baker and colleagues[17] recommend the use of a two-stage melolabial flap in order not to violate the nose-cheek junction and alar-facial sulcus. A two-stage melolabial flap is an interpolated flap with a pedicle that is generally detached after 2 to 3 weeks. Melolabial flaps are versatile and usually provide abundant skin for nasal reconstruction; however, they mainly have a random pattern vascularization, which may endanger the viability of flap in patients who have a history of radiotherapy or smoking.

Forehead Flap

Historically, the first records of forehead flaps were stated in the Indian medical literature; however, many modifications and refinements have been reported since then.[18] It is a time-honored surgical technique of nasal reconstruction and can be successfully used for the reconstruction of large and full-thickness nasal defects that are located throughout the nose. Traditionally, forehead flaps are mainly subdivided as median or paramedian according to the location of the donor site and design of flap. The paramedian forehead flap has functional and aesthetic advantages because of the easy mode of transfer and axial blood supply. The flap should be designed with a narrow pedicle to allow a wide arc of rotation with less kinking of the pedicle compared with a midline forehead flap. However, the vascularity of the pedicle should also be preserved; therefore, an ideal pedicle should be 1 to 1.5 cm in width. Some authors suggest use of Doppler ultrasonography for the detection of the supratrochlear artery, which provides the dominant blood supply to the flap; however, the authors believe that Doppler ultrasonography is only occasionally necessary, instead using anatomic landmarks to design the flap.[19–21]

Full-Thickness Nasal Defects

In full-thickness nasal defects, three-layer (inner lining, framework, and outer covering) reconstruction of the nose is essential (Fig. 2). The inner lining should be restored in order not to get flap contracture or necrosis. A myriad of surgical techniques have been suggested for the reconstruction of the inner lining. The most popular surgical techniques are intranasal lining flaps (bipedicle vestibular skin advancement flap, ipsilateral/contralateral/bilateral septal mucoperichondrial hinge flaps, septal chondromucosal pivotal flaps, turbinate mucoperiosteal flaps); buccal mucosal flaps; skin-cartilage composite grafts; turnover flaps; melolabial flaps; forehead flaps; and free flaps.[22–24] An ideal reconstructive technique should be robust of vascular supply, compliant for transfer, and thin enough not to cause nasal obstruction. Therefore, intranasal

lining flaps, especially septal mucoperichondrial flaps, are generally suggested as the first reconstructive option, if remaining healthy mucosa is adequate. The inner lining of the alar region can be re-established using ipsilateral anteriorly based septal mucoperichondrial hinge flaps. In this technique, a cul-de-sac is inevitably created that is generally separated from the septum after 2 to 3 weeks. This flap requires structural support to form the framework and avoid alar collapse or distortion. Therefore, auricular cartilage grafting, best fitted for alar contouring, is usually performed for structural support. In patients who have full-thickness nasal defects involving alar region and nasal sidewall, a combined application of ipsilateral anteriorly and contralateral superiorly based septal mucoperichondrial hinge flaps is required.[25] In these cases, the framework can be restored using auricular cartilage and quadrangular cartilage that can be harvested during the preparation of the contralateral superiorly based septal mucoperichondrial hinge flap. Indeed, care should be taken not to violate the L-strut structure of the nose by preserving adequate cartilage.

The use of full-thickness skin grafts for inner lining was popularized by Menick,[26] who introduced a three-stage forehead flap reconstruction. He combines full-thickness skin grafts with a forehead flap in the first operation and performs the structural cartilage grafting in the second operation, if necessary. Moreover, Keck and colleagues[27] reported that combined application of skin-cartilage composite grafts (inner lining and framework) and local nasal or regional flaps (outer covering) for the reconstruction of partial nasal defects provides good functional and aesthetic outcomes. In extensive loss of inner lining, forehead/melolabial flaps can also be performed, although they are generally preferred for outer covering because of their bulkiness. In addition, in cases of near-total nasal reconstruction, two separate forehead flaps can be designed for the reconstruction of inner lining and outer covering of the nose and the framework of nasal dorsum can be reconstituted using costal cartilages.[25]

Total or Near Total Reconstruction

When a near-total or total reconstruction of inner lining is required, a microvascular thin free flap, such as the radial forearm flap, is the best surgical option. Moore and colleagues[28] presented three cases of total or near-total nasal reconstruction using radial forearm free flap (inner lining); costal cartilage (framework); and paramedian forehead flap (outer covering). Although they had satisfactory outcomes, they emphasized that free flap

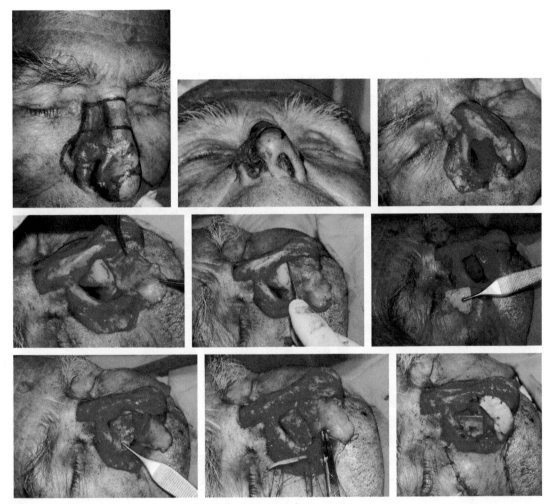

Fig. 2. Three-layer reconstruction of full-thickness nasal defect.

transfer for inner lining should be considered as the last option because of its bulkiness and donor site morbidity.

RECONSTRUCTION OF THE LIP

The lip is a complex anatomic structure and very important in terms of function and cosmesis. It plays a critical role in facial expression, kissing, sucking, oral competence, eating, drinking, deglutition, phonation, pronounciation, and speaking. The lips are bordered superiorly by the nasal base, laterally by the nasolabial sulcus, and inferiorly by the labiomental crease.

Embryologically, the upper lip is formed by the fusion of median nasal process with two maxillary processes and an intermaxillary segment; however, the lower lip is formed by the union of two mandibular processes. In an aesthetic sense, the upper lip is subdivided into three subunits by the philtrum; however, the lower lip is accepted as a single aesthetic unit. The cross-sectional anatomy of upper and lower lip is composed of four layers: (1) skin, (2) subcutaneous tissue, (3) muscle, and (4) oral mucosa. The skin forms the outer covering of the lip except the vermillion, which represents the junction of oral mucosa and outer skin. The vermillion is composed of modified mucosa, which is devoid of sweat glands, hair follicles, and minor salivary glands. In an anthropometric study, the width of the vermillion border was measured on average to be 70 mm in women and 75 mm in men.[29] It is of great cosmetic importance; any distortion or displacement of the vermillion border can easily be recognized and lead to a poor aesthetic outcome. The major muscle of the lip is the orbicularis oris muscle, which forms the bulkiness of the lip and acts as a sphincter by enfolding the mouth circularly. The arterial blood supply to the lip is derived from the branches of facial artery (lower lip, inferior labial artery; upper lip, superior labial artery). The sensory innervation

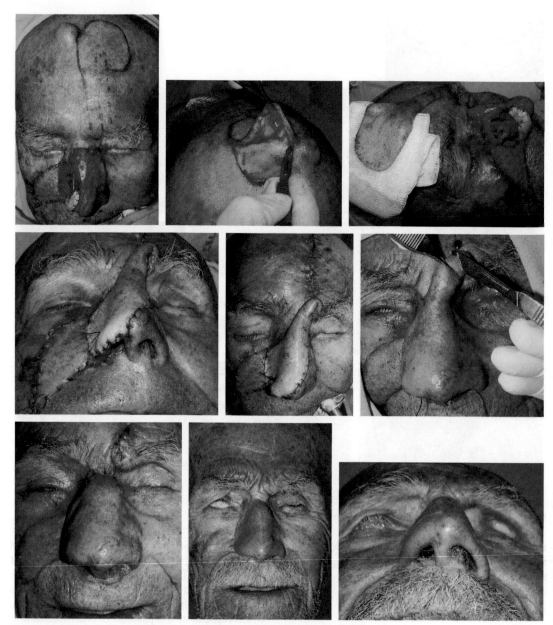

Fig. 2. (*Continued*). Three-layer reconstruction of full-thickness nasal defect.

of the lower lip is supplied by the mental nerve, a branch of mandibular division of trigeminal nerve; the sensory innervation of the upper lip is supplied by the infraorbital nerve, a branch of maxillary division of the trigeminal nerve. The motor nerve supply to the muscles of lips is buccal and marginal mandibular branches of the facial nerve.

The major goals of lip reconstruction are:

- Avoidance of microstomia
- Restoration of oral competence
- Preservation of cutaneous sensation
- Maximizing cosmesis

Every reconstruction should be tailored individually and the surgical technique should be selected according to the defect size, location, and thickness (**Fig. 3**). Therefore, lip defects can be grouped as cutaneous only; vermillion-mucosa only; or full-thickness (less than one-half, one-half to two-thirds, total or near-total).[30]

Cutaneous-Only Defects

Small defects of the lip that are limited to cutaneous and subcutaneous tissue can be reconstructed by primary closure parallel to the

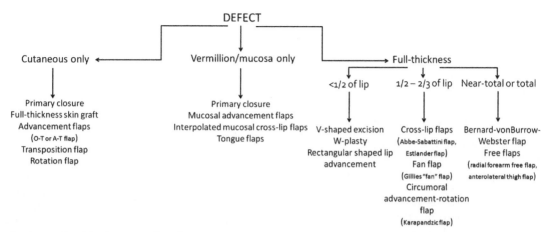

Fig. 3. An algorithmic approach to lip reconstruction.

relaxed skin tension lines. Defects that are close to the vermilion border can be repaired using A-T or O-T horizontal advancement flaps, if possible. The moderate to large cutaneous defects of the upper lip are generally reconstructed using transposition or rotation melolabial flaps. However, the reconstruction of moderate-to-large cutaneous defects of the lower lip can be accomplished using transposition or rotation flaps from chin or cheek.

Vermillion-Mucosa–Only Defects

These types of defects are generally created after vermilionectomy that is indicated for actinic cheilitis, dysplasia, and carcinoma in situ. Vermilionectomy is performed by excision of diseased mucosa of the lip down to the level of the orbicularis oris muscle. The surgical techniques for the reconstruction of vermilion defects are (1) primary closure, (2) mucosal advancement flaps, (3) interpolated mucosal cross-lip flaps, and (4) tongue flaps.[31]

Primary closure of vermilion defects is the easiest surgical technique to execute; however, it can only be applied to small mucosal defects. A mucosal advancement flap is executed by undermining the healthy adjacent remaining mucosal tissue and extending the dissection to the gingivolabial sulcus, if necessary. Thereafter, the flap is redraped over the orbicularis oris muscle and attached to the vermilion border. It is easy to perform with excellent aesthetic outcome. Nevertheless, wound contraction may cause the distortion of vermillion. Sand and colleagues[32] evaluated and compared the functional and aesthetic outcome of primary closure and mucosal advancement flaps for reconstruction of vermilion defects. They reported that mucosal advancement flaps provided better functional

and aesthetic outcome, although causing longer surgery time.

Interpolated cross-lip mucosal flaps are used to repair the larger vermilion defects by undermining and elevating an appropriate amount of mucosa and some soft tissue from the donor lip. The flap is transferred and sutured to the defect area. They can be designed as either single or bipedicled according to the amount of mucosal tissue that is necessary. The most important disadvantages of this method are that it requires a second surgery for inset of the flap after 2 to 3 weeks and restriction of certain foods is generally necessary not to violate the flap pedicle.

Tongue flaps are designed by excision of some amount of mucosal and soft tissue from the ventral or lateral side of the tongue. Although tongue flaps may provide a good color and texture match, they have similar disadvantages of interpolated cross-lip mucosal flaps. Therefore, they are generally reserved for excessive mucosal or combined mucosa-muscle defects in which bulkiness is also required.

Full-Thickness Defects

Full-thickness lip defects should be reconstructed in four layers: (1) skin, (2) subcutaneous tissue, (3) muscle, and (4) oral mucosa. Whenever possible the continuity of orbicularis oris muscle should be re-established. In an aesthetic sense, the vermillion border should be formed without any distortion or displacement. The surgical techniques that are used in the reconstruction of full-thickness lip defects can be grouped as:

1. Reconstruction using the remaining lip tissue: wedge-shaped excision, W-shaped excision, and lip advancement flaps

2. Reconstruction with transfer or rotation of tissue from the healthy lip: Abbe-Sabattini flap, Estlander flap, Gillies fan flap, and Karapandzic flap
3. Reconstruction with recruitment of adjacent cheek tissue: Bernard-von Burow-Webster flap
4. Reconstruction with free flaps: Radial forearm free flap, anterolateral thigh flap

The surgical techniques for reconstruction of full-thickness defects of the lip are generally selected according to the size of the defect area. They are classified into three groups: (1) full-thickness defects involving one-half of the lip, (2) full-thickness defects involving one-half to two-thirds of the lip, and (3) near-total and total lip defects.

Full-thickness defects involving one-half of the lip

Full-thickness defects involving up to 30% of the transverse width of the lip can be reconstructed using primary closure, which does not usually lead to microstomia.[33,34] When excising lip tissue, the incisions should be designed according to the relaxed skin tension lines; and the terminal angle at the vertex should be around 30 degrees. A classic V-shaped excision is generally suggested for medially localized tumor excision; however, a "lazy" V-shaped excision generally provides a better aesthetic outcome for laterally localized defects. If the apex of incisions extends or passes the mentolabial crease or nasolabial sulcus, a W-shaped excision is preferred in order not to violate the chin or cheek. In this case, both apexes of the incisions should not exceed 30 degrees.

Full-thickness defects that are larger than one-third and smaller than one-half of the width of the lip can be reconstructed by lip advancement flaps, which are generally designed as rectangular-shaped.

Full-thickness defects involving one-half to two-thirds of the lip

Full-thickness defects involving more than one-half of the width of the lip cannot be reconstructed by simple advancement of the remaining lip elements; therefore, tissue borrowing is necessary. The major surgical techniques that are especially preferred for these defects are cross-lip flaps (Abbe-Sabattini flap and Estlander flap); fan flap (Gillies "fan" flap); and circumoral advancement-rotation flaps (Karapandzic flap).

The cross-lip flaps are designed by creating a full-thickness lip flap from the opposite lip. The width of the flap should be one-half of the width of the defect; thereby, the width of both lips is equalized. In addition, the width of the flap should not exceed 2 cm. The arterial blood of the flap is supplied by the labial artery (either superior or inferior); therefore, full-thickness incisions of the cross-lip flap should be performed without injuring the labial arteries, which are located just below the vermillion border. Thereafter, the flap is rotated and attached to the defect area and the donor site is closed primarily. The most important advantages of these flaps are that defects can be reconstructed by most like tissue and continuity of muscle fibers can be maintained. Cross-lip flaps are technically subdivided into two as the Abbe-Sabattini flap and the Estlander flap. The Abbe-Sabattini flap is a two-staged procedure especially used for defects not including the commissure. The pedicle can be detached after 2 to 3 weeks. The main drawbacks of the Abbe-Sabattini flap are potential risk of vermilion misalignment and lip adhesion. The Estlander flap is preferred for the defects including the commissure. Although it is a single-stage procedure, commissureplasty is generally required because of distortion.

Gillie "fan" flap is a modification of the Estlander flap, which is principally formed by the recruitment of the ipsilateral remaining lip elements with more tissue from the nasolabial region and opposing lip. A unilateral Gillie "fan" flap is best suited for moderate-to-large lip defects. Bilateral Gillie "fan" flaps can also be performed for near-total defects of lip; however, microstomia, vermilion misalignment, and rounded commissures are inevitable. In addition, a reversible denervation generally occurs and may lead to oral incompetence, although the continuity of orbicularis oris muscle is mostly preserved.[35]

The Karapandzic flap is an advancement-rotation flap in which the lip is reconstructed by innervated orbicularis oris muscle with decreasing the total circumference (**Fig. 4**). In this flap, curved circumoral incisions are performed in or parallel to the nasolabial sulcus. Thereby, remaining and opposing lip tissue is mobilized and repositioned to re-establish the lip. The key issue is to preserve the neurovascular bundle and blood supply, which is primarily based on the superior and inferior labial arteries. The most important disadvantage of this flap is the potential risk of microstomia and blunting of the oral commissure. Hanasono and Langstein[36] suggested a modification of the Karapandzic flap in which the flaps are extended by recruiting adjacent tissue from the perioral cheek. They advocated that this modification may allow reconstruction of near-total and total lower lip defects without causing microstomia.

Near-total and total lip defects

Near-total or total lip reconstruction is a challenging issue in which remaining lip tissue is

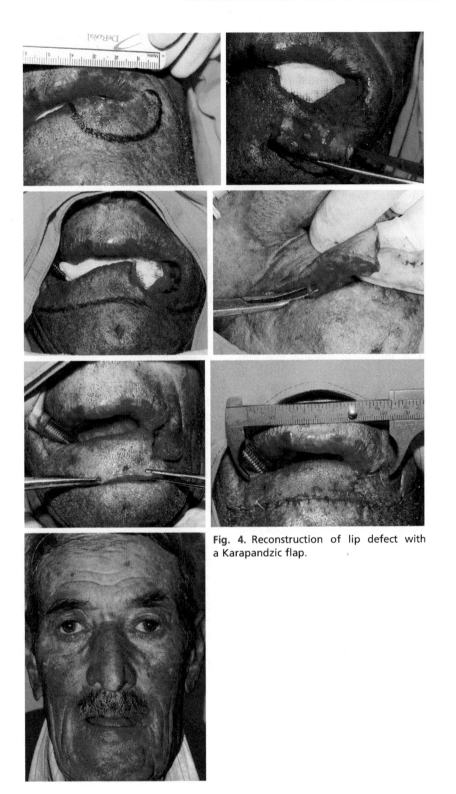

Fig. 4. Reconstruction of lip defect with a Karapandzic flap.

insufficient; besides, the defect may involve adjacent units, such as nose, cheek, and chin. Therefore, a significant amount of tissue borrowing is always required from regional tissues, which can be recruited from cheek or distant tissues that can be derived by free flaps.

The Bernard-von Burrow-Webster flap is a regional flap especially preferred for near-total or total lip reconstruction. It is designed by advancing remaining lip and bilateral cheek tissue. In this flap, cheek tissue and remaining lip tissue are recruited together and attached in the midline. Multiple Burrow triangles are excised to mobilize the cheek tissue. The laxity of the cheek is a key issue for a successful flap design; therefore, this must be evaluated preoperatively. In this technique, adding cheek tissue reduces the incidence of microstomia. However, transfer of static tissue may lead to oral incompetence and drooling.[30]

Free flaps are the mainstay for near-total and total lip reconstruction. The most frequently preferred flap is the radial forearm free flap, because it is easy to harvest, has a long pedicle, and has appropriate vessel caliber with reasonable color and texture match. In addition, it has a thin and pliable skin paddle, which provides adequate tissue to restore the mucosa and skin elements of the lip simultaneously. The blood supply of the radial forearm free flap is primarily based on the radial artery. Although it is a fasciocutaneous flap, palmaris longus tendon can also be included, if it is present. Palmaris longus tendon can be attached to the remaining orbicularis oris muscle; thereby, a partially dynamic closure of the oral stoma can be achieved. Carroll and colleagues[37] (10 patients), Özdemir and colleagues[38] (17 patients), and Jeng and colleagues[39] (12 patients) reported successful reconstruction of near-total and total lip defects using radial forearm-palmaris longus tendon-free flaps. They emphasized that good functional outcome (especially oral competence) and satisfactory aesthetic outcome can be achieved by this technique. In addition, aesthetic outcome can be improved by further refinements, such as mucosal grafts, tongue flaps, vermilion tattooing, fat injections, or defatting.[40]

RECONSTRUCTION OF THE CHEEK

The cheek is the largest aesthetic unit of the face and has contiguities with crucial midface structures, such as orbita, nose, and lip. Its boundaries are lateral margin of the nose and nasolabial sulcus medially, the infraorbital rim and zygomatic arch superiorly, preauricular crease laterally, and lower border of the mandible inferiorly. It also contains vital anatomic structures, such as branches of facial nerve and Stensen duct. Roth and colleagues[41] subdivide the cheek into three zones according to skin laxity, texture, and mobility: zone 1, infraorbital and perioral medial cheek region; zone 2, preauricular region; and zone 3, buccomandibular region.

In the infraorbital region, the skin laxity is relatively less and inappropriately designed flaps may lead to eyelid complications, such as ectropion. In the preauricular region, the redundancy of skin is greater, especially in geriatric patients; therefore, most of the defects that are localized to zone 2 can often be reconstructed by primary closure. The buccomandibular region is the largest aesthetic subunit of the cheek and often has adequate skin to allow reconstruction with local flaps. Through-and-through defects of the buccal region should be restored in three layers: (1) oral mucosa, (2) volumetric filling for bulkiness, and (3) skin. The major goals of cheek reconstruction are to obtain a functioning and aesthetically normal-appearing cheek with minimal scars.

Surgical techniques used for cheek reconstruction include primary closure, skin grafting, local and regional flaps, and free flaps (Fig. 5). Most partial-thickness cheek defects can be reconstructed by one of these methods. However, free flaps are generally required for reconstruction of near-total/total and large full-thickness cheek defects.

Primary Closure

Primary closure is the ideal surgical technique for repair of small-to-moderate sized partial-thickness cheek defects. To maximize the aesthetic outcome, surgeons should attempt to convert the shape of the defect to a fusiform configuration, if possible. The incisions of fusiform excision should be oriented parallel to the curvilinear relaxed skin tension lines and hidden in native creases and aesthetic boundary lines. Thereafter, subcutaneous tissue is undermined. However, undermining around the upper lip and lower eyelid should be performed carefully not to cause tissue distortion, such as misalignment of vermilion or ectropion. When the defect is located at the periphery of the cheek, an elliptical closure with M-plasty can shorten the length of the closure line and may be preferred.[42,43] In a retrospective study, Rapstine and colleagues[44] reported that more than half of their patients who underwent reconstruction of cheek because of tumor resection had successful primary wound closure. They also emphasized that the redundancy of cheek skin provides sufficient skin with an excellent

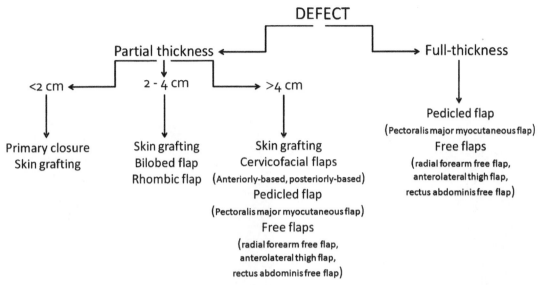

Fig. 5. An algorithmic approach to cheek reconstruction.

vascular supply to minimize scarring and ensure an acceptable aesthetic outcome.

Skin Grafting

Skin grafting of cheek defects is rarely preferred because of patchy appearance and poor color and texture match between the graft and the adjacent cheek skin. However, full-thickness skin grafting can be used for large cheek defects that are localized to zone 1, especially around the orbital margin. In addition, skin grafting may be performed in cases when excision of skin cancer involves surgical margins that are unreliable for the presence of persistent tumor.

Local and Regional Flaps

Local flaps are the preferred surgical technique for the reconstruction of small-to-moderate partial-thickness cheek defects. Although all types of local flaps can be used, bilobed and rhombic flaps are the most preferred because of their geometry. In addition, cervicofacial flaps are the workhorse for the reconstruction of large partial-thickness cheek defects.

Bilobed flap

The bilobed flap is a modified rotation and transposition flap with a precise geometric design (**Fig. 6**). These flaps are best suited for repair of defects where there is insufficient skin redundancy in the immediate area of the defect to create a flap for wound closure. Although the original design of the bilobe flap was initially described by Esser in 1918, many modifications have been reported

thereafter. The authors generally prefer the following technique: two lobes (the first lobe is approximately equal to the defect area and the second lobe is two thirds of the defect area) are harvested from two donor sites separated by an angle of 45 degrees. The height of the second lobe is lengthened for primary closure of its donor defect.

Rhombic flap

There are many modifications of the rhombic flap, but the most popular designs are the Limberg and Dufourmental flaps. The Limberg flap is formed as equilateral parallelograms with interior angles of 60 and 120 degrees and can be designed in four different orientations. Chu and Byrne[45] noted that the orientation of the flap should be determined according to the areas of skin laxity and tension, and the relaxed skin tension lines or aesthetic borders.

Cervicofacial flap

Cervicofacial flaps are locoregional advancement-rotation flaps in which skin from cheek, neck, and even chest are used for the reconstruction of large cheek defects. They can be harvested anteriorly or posteriorly based according to the flap design. Anteriorly based cervicofacial flaps are especially useful for large anterior cheek defects; however, posteriorly based cervicofacial flaps are generally preferred for small-to-moderate sized anterior cheek defects.[45–47] One of the most important advantages of these flaps in reconstruction of large cheek defects is the use of neck skin, which has an excellent skin color and texture match with the skin of the cheek. In addition, scarring is generally

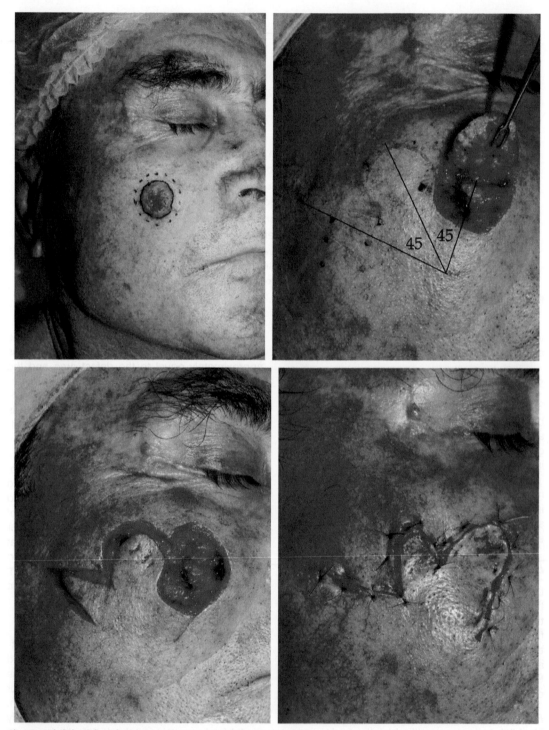

Fig. 6. A bilobed flap for the reconstruction of cheek defect.

inconspicuous with an acceptable aesthetic outcome when the incisions are placed in natural creases or aesthetic borders.[43] However, the drawbacks of these flaps are ectropion, hematoma, or seroma and flap necrosis. Ectropion generally occurs because of downward pull of flap tissue in the area of the lower eyelid. The surgeon should make every effort to minimize wound closure tension in the area of the lower eyelid. This can sometimes be achieved by designing the incision

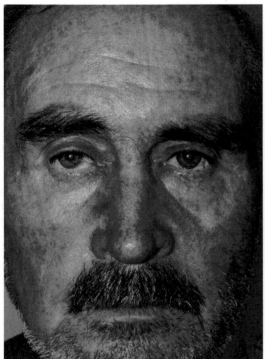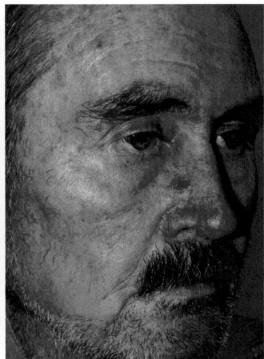

Fig. 6. (*Continued*). Postoperative outcome of bilobed flap for the reconstruction of cheek defect.

above the lateral canthus in the temporal area or suspending the flap to the lateral orbit when using this flap to reconstruct upper medial cheek defects. Hematomas can be prevented by executing meticulous hemostatis during surgery, placing drains and using topical hemostatic agents, if necessary. Flap necrosis is usually partial or at the distal border of the flap and may occur in extensively mobilized random pattern cervicofacial flaps. The risk of flap necrosis is remarkably increased in patients who have ischemic problems caused by diabetes, history of smoking, or radiation.

Cervicofacial flaps can be elevated as a random skin and subcutaneous tissue flap or deep-plane composite flap. Subcutaneous cervicofacial skin flaps are easy to harvest with a lower risk of facial nerve injury than composite flaps; however, the blood supply is less. In contrast, deep-plane cervicofacial flaps are elevated below the superficial musculoaponeurotic system and have an improved vascular supply. However, the elevation of such flaps is technically difficult with higher risk of facial nerve injury. A deep plane cervicofacial flap is suggested for patients having a high risk of flap necrosis to enhance the flap reliability by maximizing the blood supply to the flap.[48,49] Austen and colleagues[50] retrospectively evaluated 32 patients who underwent a subcutaneous cerviofacial flap to repair large cheek defects. In this study, only minor ectropion was detected in one

case and distal necrosis of the margin of the flap was detected in three cases. They believe that the surgical success of subcutaneous cervicofacial flaps is comparable with deep plane cervicofacial flaps, and the risk of damage to vital structures, such as the facial nerve, is less.

Myocutaneous flap

The pectoralis major myocutaneous flap is occasionally used to reconstruct very large cheek defects. It is a surgical option in cases where the bulkiness of the flap is useful in providing large amounts of subcutaneous soft tissue. In a retrospective study, McLean and colleagues[51] reported that they successfully use this flap to reconstruct 24 patients with temporal or cheek defects; however, the aesthetic outcome was not evaluated in this study. In addition, Ahmad and colleagues[52] has used pectoralis major myocutaneous flaps designed with two skin islands for the reconstruction of full-thickness cheek defects. They emphasized that although it is not the first option for these defects, this technique can be useful when free flaps are not applicable or free flap failure has occurred.

Free Flaps

Large and full-thickness defects of the cheek are challenging, because at least two-layer reconstruction (internal lining [oral mucosa] and outer covering [skin]) is necessary. In these cases, free flaps are usually the preferred method of reconstruction and involve the microsurgical transfer of tissue to the deficits of oral mucosa and skin simultaneously. The ideal free flap for the reconstruction of full-thickness defects of the cheek is the radial forearm free flap; however, the anterolateral thigh and rectus abdominis free flap can also be used. Two skin paddles are harvested as part of the radial forearm free flap, which is then folded on itself to provide internal and external replacement of missing tissue. Radial forearm free flaps are easy to harvest with a long pedicle and have blood vessels of large caliber; therefore, they can be easily anastomosed to the facial artery and vein. In addition, the donor site morbidity is low and cosmetic outcomes are acceptable. Recently, the anterolateral thigh free flap designed as a fasciocutaneous or musculocutaneous flap has been popularized for the reconstruction of full-thickness defects of the cheek. The flap is based on lateral circumflex femoral artery. Ozkan and colleagues[53] reported 24 patients who underwent successful reconstruction of buccal defects using the anterolateral thigh free flap. They stated that the anterolateral thigh free flap is reliable and when used for the repair of buccal defects results in an excellent functional and aesthetic outcome.

RECONSTRUCTION OF THE FOREHEAD

The forehead is a well-vascularized flat region of the face. It makes up a single aesthetic facial unit and its boundaries are hairline superiorly and laterally, and glabella, eyebrows, and supraorbital rim inferiorly. The forehead is divided into four regions: (1) central, (2) paramedian, (3) temporal, and (4) glabellar. The major goals of forehead reconstruction are (1) to preserve the motor (frontal branch of facial nerve) and sensory (supraorbital and supratrochlear branch of trigeminal nerve) innervation; (2) to cause minimal irregularities or misalignment at the eyebrows and hairline; and (3) to camouflage the incisions and scars in the natural borders, such as hairline and eyebrow, or natural creases, such as rhytids.

The surgical techniques for forehead reconstruction are dependent on the vertical, transverse, and anteroposterior skin laxity and the location of the defect. Reconstructive options for forehead defects are healing by secondary intention, primary wound closure, skin grafting, local and regional flaps, and free flaps (**Fig. 7**).

Healing by secondary intention is the easiest procedure for forehead reconstruction. It is best suited for concave regions of the forehead, such as the temporal region. Satisfactory cosmetic outcomes can also be achieved in other regions.

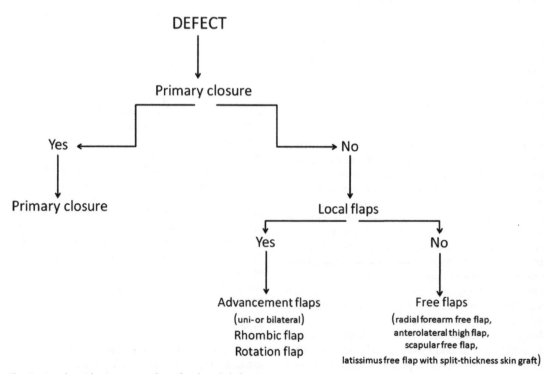

Fig. 7. An algorithmic approach to forehead defects.

Although it can be an option for any size defect, hairline or eyebrow irregularities may occur in large defects as the wound contracts. Therefore, a "purse-string" suture can be applied to decrease the size of the defect especially in large forehead defects. Meticulous wound care with antibiotic ointments is required for weeks to months before healing is complete.

Primary wound closure is the preferred method of repair if tissue is sufficient. Small-to-moderate defects (<3 cm) especially located in the central portion of the forehead can be successfully reconstructed by primary closure. The defect is transformed into a fusiform shape and vertically designed incisions are generally preferred in order not to distort the eyebrow. Wide undermining should be performed for tension-free closure. A W-plasty or M-plasty can be performed if a standing cutaneous deformity requires excision. Subcutaneous dissection is adequate for small defects; however, dissection beneath the fascia is required for larger defects. In this case, the frontal branch of facial nerve, which courses beneath the frontalis muscle, is at risk in the temporal region and care is taken in this area of dissection.

Skin grafting is occasionally used to repair forehead defects, but results in a poor skin color and texture match with adjacent forehead skin. Nevertheless, it can be used in patients who have granulation tissue caused by healing by secondary intention; thereby, the duration of wound healing can be shortened.

Advancement and rotation flaps are commonly used for forehead reconstruction. Unilateral and bilateral horizontal advancement flaps are useful when skin laxity is not sufficient or forehead defects are too large to close primarily. These flaps respect the eyebrows and hairline, when they are properly designed along relaxed skin tension lines. Aesthetic outcomes of these flaps are excellent, if incisions are placed in the forehead rhytids. The O-T flap and A-T flap are modifications of advancement flaps that are especially preferred when a border of the defect is close to the hairline or eyebrow[54] (**Fig. 8**). They minimize misalignment of the eyebrow or hairline. Rotation flaps are best suited for moderate-sized forehead defects that are located in the lateral and paramedian forehead regions. Although there are many design modifications, the Worthen rotation flap is the mainstay for large forehead defects. The most important limitations of rotation flaps are elevation of the eyebrow, pincushion deformity, and suboptimal aesthetic outcome caused by long curvilinear scars.

A tissue expander can be used and placed adjacent or closed to the defect area, when the defect area is very large (>6 cm). However, the reconstruction must be staged in this case and performed at least 3 to 4 weeks after the skin cancer excision. Therefore, some authors prefer the use of free flaps, such as the radial forearm or anterolateral thigh flap. McCombe and coworkers[55] reported 29 patients who underwent free flap transfer to the forehead or scalp after excision of skin cancer. They emphasized that locally advanced skin cancers of the forehead and scalp can be successfully reconstructed by free flaps and aesthetic outcome can be improved by refinement surgeries. Beasley and coworkers[56] recommended a staging system for the selection of a reconstructive surgical technique depending on the defect size. This staging system includes four groups: (IA) defects involving less than half of the surface area of the forehead, (IB) defects involving less than half of the surface area of the forehead with osteomyelitis or osteroradionecrosis, (II) defects that are more than half of the surface area of the forehead, and (III) defects more than half of the surface area of the forehead extending into the scalp. They recommended that IA forehead defects can be reconstructed by primary closure or local flaps, IB and II forehead defects can be reconstructed with a scapular free flap, and III forehead defects can be reconstructed with a scapular free flap or latissimus free flap and split-thickness skin grafts. Van Driel and colleagues[57] suggested an algorithm for the microvascular reconstruction of complex forehead or scalp defects. According to this algorithm, the defects that are limited to the forehead can be reconstructed by thin fasciocutaneous flaps, such as the radial forearm, parascapular, or anterolateral thigh free flaps. However, a muscle flap with thick skin graft, such as the latissimus dorsi or rectus abdominis free flap, is preferred for immediate reconstruction, when the defect involves forehead and another facial unit.

RECONSTRUCTION OF THE EYELID

The upper and lower eyelids have a complex anatomic structure with eight different layers:

1. Skin
2. Subcutaneous tissue
3. Orbicularis oculi muscle
4. Orbital septum
5. Fat tissue
6. Müller and levator muscles for upper eyelid, capsulopalpebral fascia, and inferior tarsal muscle for lower eyelid
7. Tarsus
8. Conjunctiva

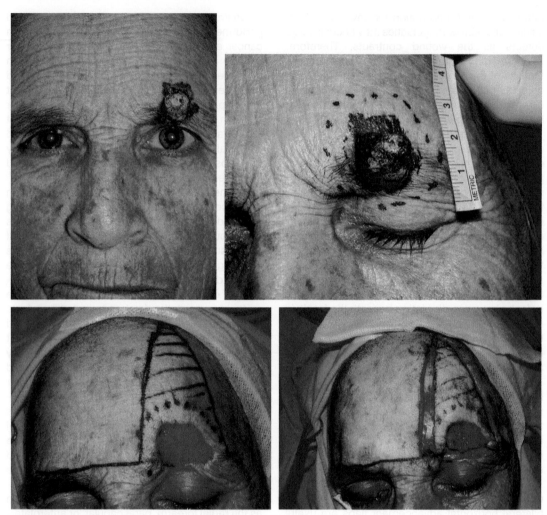

Fig. 8. Reconstruction of forehead defect with an A-T flap.

In addition, the eyelids are divided into two surgical units: anterior skin-muscle lamella and posterior tarso-conjuctival lamella. The posterior lamella directly contacts the ocular surfaces and the anterior lamella forms the outer covering. Both eyelids work as a unit to preserve the integrity of cornea and protect and support the eye. Any defect of the eyelids, especially upper eyelid, may lead to corneal abrasions and erosions if proper reconstruction is not performed. The surgical technique for reconstruction of the upper and lower eyelid mainly depends on the size and thickness of the defect, eyelid laxity, and availability of surrounding tissues (**Fig. 9**).

Primary closure is generally possible for defects that involve less than 20% to 33% of the width of the upper or lower eyelid. It can provide the most optimal functional and aesthetic outcome. Anterior lamella defects can generally be closed in fusiform fashion by nonabsorbable sutures, such as 6/0 silk sutures. However, full-thickness defects are usually converted to a pentagonal shape and a three-layer closure performed. Initially, the tarsal plate is reapproximated with absorbable sutures, such as 6/0 vicryl suture; lid margin sutures are placed reciprocally (gray line to gray line, lash line to lash line, mucocutaneous junction to mucocutaneous junction) with nonabsorbable sutures, such as 6/0 silk suture; and finally skin is approximated with 6/0 silk suture. Moreover, a lateral canthotomy or cantholysis can be performed when excessive wound tension occurs.

Grafts may play a critical role for the reconstruction of anterior and posterior lamella defects of upper and lower eyelids. Full-thickness skin grafts are useful for the reconstruction of defects that involve only the anterior lamella of the eyelids. The redundant skin of ipsilateral or contralateral upper

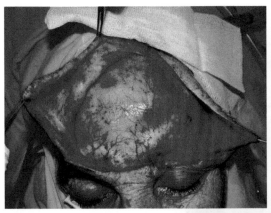
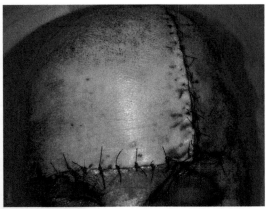
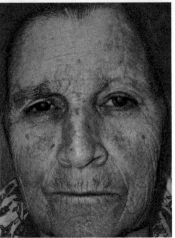

Fig. 8. (*Continued*). Reconstruction of forehead defect with an A-T flap and outcome.

eyelid is best suited as a donor site for the skin graft and provides the best color and texture match. However, preauricular and postauricular and supraclavicular regions can also be used as an alternative donor site. Posterior lamella defects of the eyelids can be reconstructed using grafts of tarsoconjunctiva, buccal mucosa, hard palate mucosa, or nasal septal mucoperichondrium with or without cartilage. Autogenous tarsoconjunctival grafts can be obtained from the contralateral upper eyelid and provides the best option for the reconstruction of posterior lamella.[58] However, the major drawback is the limited amount of graft tissue that can be harvested. Buccal or labial mucosa is a reliable source of grafts for repair of posterior lamella defects of eyelids. Whitehouse and Francis[59] performed a combined buccal mucosa graft and myocutaneous flap successfully to repair 15 patients with full-thickness defects of the eyelids. They emphasized that this is an easy, one-stage procedure that allows good tissue match. They noted that palatal mucosal grafts are also a satisfactory substitute for the posterior lamella of the tarsus and conjunctiva in eyelid reconstruction. They include mucosa and

periosteum, thereby providing a smooth surface and structural support to the graft. Some authors report excessive irritation of the cornea when palatal grafts are used.[60] Nevertheless, Tanaka and colleagues[61] and Ito and colleagues[62] reported successful management of posterior lamella defects of the upper eyelid with palatal mucosal grafts. Nasal septal mucoperichondrium is also an option for the reconstruction of the posterior lamella. Moreover, composite septal cartilage-mucoperichondrium grafts can be harvested to enhance support when reconstructing the lower eyelid.

Cutler-Beard Flap

Moderate and large posterior lamellar defects of the upper eyelid can be reconstructed by a sliding tarsoconjunctival flap or Cutler-Beard flap (bridge flap). The sliding tarsoconjunctival flap is designed from the residual adjacent healthy lid tissue. In this technique, the tarsoconjunctival tissue of the flap is advanced horizontally to close the posterior lamella defect. Although it is easy to perform, its

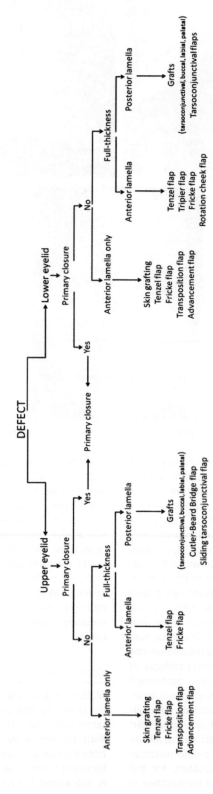

Fig. 9. An algorithmic approach to eyelid reconstruction.

use is limited by the amount of remaining tarsal plate available for reconstruction. In addition, lid retraction, lid margin deformity, lack of cilia, and abnormal lid contour may occur.

The Cutler-Beard flap is a two-stage procedure especially useful for the reconstruction of large posterior lamellar defects of the upper eyelid. It is performed by creating a full-thickness (cutaneo-myo-conjunctival) lower lid flap, which is transferred to the upper eyelid defect. This technique does not allow the reconstruction of the tarsal plate, which may cause cicatricial entropion or eyelid contraction; therefore, a cartilage graft is generally required. The pedicle of the flap is detached after 2 to 3 weeks.

Tarsoconjunctival Flaps

Moderate-to-large posterior lamella defects of the lower eyelid can be reconstructed by advancement tarsoconjunctival flaps (modified Hughes procedure). The modified Hughes procedure is a two-stage surgery in which a part of posterior lamellar tissue is borrowed from the upper eyelid. It is designed as a vascularized flap from the upper eyelid conjunctiva and tarsus. At least 4 mm of upper tarsus along the lid margin is preserved to ensure the stability of the upper eyelid. The remaining superior conjunctiva and tarsus is elevated and transferred to the posterior lamellar defect of the lower eyelid. The tarsal margins of the tarsoconjunctival flap are attached to the remaining tarsal edges of the lower eyelid defect using absorbable sutures, such as 6/0 vicryl sutures. Eye closure for at least 2 weeks is the major drawback of this procedure.

Rotational Flaps

Moderate to large (30%–60%) anterior lamellar defects of the eyelids can be reconstructed by semicircular-shaped rotational flaps (Tenzel flap) or Fricke flap. The Tenzel flap is a semicircular rotational skin-muscle flap that is designed from the adjacent skin beyond the lateral canthus. The technique is useful for upper and lower eyelid reconstruction, although they are designed in a different fashion. An inferior arching superiorly based flap incision for upper eyelid defects and a superior arching inferiorly based flap incision for lower eyelid are used.[60] The superior crus (for upper eyelid) or inferior crus (for inferior eyelid) of the lateral canthal tendon is identified and separated from its attachment at the orbital rim after a lateral canthotomy. The flap should be raised in a suborbicularis plane up to the orbital rim and subcutaneously thereafter, thereby reducing the risk of injury to the zygomatic branch of facial

nerve. The lateral part of the eyelid is mobilized medially together with the skin flap and the wound closure is sutured under minimal tension. The flap is attached to the inner periosteum of the lateral orbital rim, which prevents the sagging of flap caused by gravity.

Temporal Flap

The Fricke flap (temporal forehead flap) can be used for near-total to total anterior lamellar defects of upper and lower eyelid. It is a laterally based transposition skin flap elevated from the suprabrow region. A subcutaneous dissection is generally preferred to avoid bulkiness of the reconstructed eyelid. In a retrospective study, the modified Fricke flap was evaluated; 15 of 20 patients reported satisfactory outcome in functional (10 excellent and 5 good) and aesthetic results (3 excellent and 12 good).[63]

Lateral or Medial Flap

The Tripier flap is a unipedicle or bipedicle laterally or medially based flap formed from upper eyelid skin, which is useful for the reconstruction of anterior lamellar defects of the lower eyelid.[64] The excess skin above the upper lid crease composes the flap together with the underlying orbicularis oculi muscle. The flap is transferred to the lower lid and sutured to the wound edges of the defect.

Cheek Rotation Flap

Mustarde cheek rotation flap is preferred for combined defects of lower eyelid and cheek.[60] The superior edge of the incision should be directed upward at the level of the lateral canthus and curve toward the preauricular region. This flap should be dissected in the subcutaneous plane over the zygomatic bone and subsuperficial musculoaponeurotic system beyond. The size of the flap should be designed three to four times the surface area of the defect; therefore, a significant amount of undermining is necessary.

SUMMARY

Facial reconstruction is a challenge from a functional and aesthetic aspect. The goal of facial reconstructive surgery is to restore anatomic integrity, preserve function, and provide an aesthetically pleasing appearance. Every facial defect that occurs after nonmelanoma skin cancer excision should be evaluated individually according to its location, size, shape, thickness, and relationships with adjacent facial structures. An accurate surgical plan should be formulated preoperatively and the most favorable surgical technique selected according to the surgeon's experience. Finally, the surgical options, likely functional and aesthetic outcomes, and potential complications should be completely discussed with the patient.

REFERENCES

1. Burget GC, Menick FJ. The subunit principle in nasal reconstruction. Plast Reconstr Surg 1985; 76:239–47.

2. Menick FJ. Artistry in aesthetic surgery. Aesthetic perception and the subunit principle. Clin Plast Surg 1987;14:723–35.

3. Rohrich RJ, Griffin JR, Ansari M, et al. Nasal reconstruction-beyond aesthetic subunits: a 15-year review of 1334 cases. Plast Reconstr Surg 2005; 114:1405–16.

4. Rodriguez-Bruno KM, Byrne PJ. Philosophy on the closing of facial defects: choosing the right procedure. Op Tech Otolaryngol 2011;22:2–12.

5. Zitelli JA. Secondary intention healing: an alternative to surgical repair. Clin Dermatol 1984;2:92–106.

6. Zitelli JA. Wound healing by secondary intention: a cosmetic appraisal. J Am Acad Dermatol 1983;9: 407–15.

7. van der Eerden PA, Lohuis PJ, Hart AA, et al. Secondary intention healing after excision of nonmelanoma skin cancer of the head and neck: statistical evaluation of prognostic values of wound characteristics and final cosmetic results. Plast Reconstr Surg 2008; 122:1747–55.

8. Jacobs MA, Christenson LJ, Weaver AL, et al. Clinical outcome of cutaneous flaps versus full-thickness skin grafts after Mohs surgery on the nose. Dermatol Surg 2010;36:23–30.

9. Jewett BS. Repair of small nasal defects. Otolaryngol Clin North Am 2007;40:337–60.

10. Baker SR. Local cutaneous flaps. Otolaryngol Clin North Am 1994;27:139–59.

11. Weber SM, Baker SR. Management of cutaneous nasal defects. Facial Plast Surg Clin North Am 2009;17:395–417.

12. Jackson I. Nose reconstruction. In: Jackson I, editor. Local flaps in head and neck reconstruction. St. Louis, Missouri: QMP Inc; 2007. p. 101–241.

13. Johnson TM, Swanson NA, Baker SR, et al. The Rieger flap for nasal reconstruction. Arch Otolaryngol Head Neck Surg 1995;121:634–7.

14. Wentzell JM. Dorsal nasal flap for reconstruction of full-thickness defects of the nose. Dermatol Surg 2010;36:1171–8.

15. Thornton JF, Weathers WM. Nasolabial flap for nasal tip reconstruction. Plast Reconstr Surg 2008;122: 775–81.

16. Fazio MJ, Zitelli JA. The single-stage nasolabial flap. Op Tech Plast Reconstr Surg 1998;5:50–8.

17. Baker SR, Johnson TM, Nelson BR. The importance of maintaining the alar-facial sulcus in nasal reconstruction. Arch Otolaryngol Head Neck Surg 1995; 121:617–22.

18. Boyd CM, Baker SR, Fader DJ, et al. The forehead flap for nasal reconstruction. Arch Dermatol 2000; 136:1365–70.

19. Yeatts RP, Newsom RW, Matthews BL. Doppler-assisted vascular pedicle flaps in eyelid and periorbital reconstruction. Arch Ophthalmol 1996;114: 1149–52.

20. Ugur MB, Savranlar A, Uzun L, et al. A reliable surface landmark for localizing supratrochlear artery: medial canthus. Otolaryngol Head Neck Surg 2008;138: 162–5.

21. Eskiizmir G, Hırçın Z, Ünlü HH. A practical method for designing paramedian forehead flap: a preliminary study. Turkiye Klinikleri J Med Sci 2010;30:1210–3.

22. Menick FJ. Lining options in nasal reconstruction. Op Tech Plast Reconstr Surg 1998;5:65–75.

23. Baker SR. Intranasal lining flaps. Op Tech Otolaryngol 2011;22:72–83.

24. Weber SM, Wang TD. Options for internal lining in nasal reconstruction. Facial Plast Surg Clin North Am 2011;19:163–73.

25. Baker SR. Reconstruction of the nose. In: Baker SR, editor. Local flaps in facial reconstruction. Philadelphia (PA): Elsevier Inc.; 2007. p. 415–75.

26. Menick FJ. The use of skin grafts for nasal lining. Clin Plast Surg 2001;28:311–21.

27. Keck T, Lindemann J, Kühnemann S, et al. Healing of composite chondrocutaneous auricular grafts covered by skin flaps in nasal reconstructive surgery. Laryngoscope 2003;113:248–53.

28. Moore EJ, Strome SA, Kasperbauer JL, et al. Vascularized radial forearm free tissue transfer for lining in nasal reconstruction. Laryngoscope 2003;113: 2078–85.

29. Ferrario VF, Rosati R, Peretta R, et al. Labial morphology: a 3-dimensional anthropometric study. J Oral Maxillofac Surg 2009;67:1832–9.

30. Coppit GL, Lin DT, Burkey BB. Current concepts in lip reconstruction. Curr Opin Otolaryngol Head Neck Surg 2004;12:281–7.

31. Renner GJ. Reconstruction of the lip. In: Baker SR, editor. Local flaps in facial reconstruction. Philadelphia (PA): Elsevier Inc.; 2007. p. 475–525.

32. Sand M, Altmeyer P, Bechara FG. Mucosal advancement flap versus primary closure after vermilionectomy of the lower lip. Dermatol Surg 2010; 36:1987–92.

33. Cupp CL, Larrabee WF. Reconstruction of the lips. Op Tech Otolaryngol Head Neck Surg 1993;4:46–53.

34. Baumann D, Robb G. Lip reconstruction. Semin Plast Surg 2008;22:269–80.

35. McCarn KE, Park SS. Lip reconstruction. Otolaryngol Clin North Am 2007;40:361–80.

36. Hanasono MM, Langstein HN. Extended Kara-pandzic flaps for near-total and total lower lip defects. Plast Reconstr Surg 2011;127:1199–205.

37. Carroll CM, Pathak I, Irish J, et al. Reconstruction of total lower lip and chin defects using the composite radial forearm–palmaris longus tendon free flap. Arch Facial Plast Surg 2000;2:53–6.

38. Ozdemir R, Ortak T, Kocer U, et al. Total lower lip reconstruction using sensate composite radial fore-arm flap. J Craniomaxillofac Surg 2003;14:393–405.

39. Jeng SF, Kuo YR, Wei FC, et al. Total lower lip recon-struction with a composite radial forearm-palmaris longus tendon flap: a clinical series. Plast Reconstr Surg 2004;113:19–23.

40. Keskin M, Sutcu M, Tosun Z, et al. Reconstruction of total lower lip defects using radial forearm free flap with subsequent tongue flap. J Craniofac Surg 2010;21:349–51.

41. Roth DA, Longaker MT, Zide BM. Cheek surface reconstruction: best choices according to zones. Op Tech Plast Reconstr Surg 1998;5:26–36.

42. Bradley DT, Murakami CS. Reconstruction of the cheek. In: Baker SR, editor. Local flaps in facial reconstruction. Phialdelphia (PA): Elsevier Inc; 2007. p. 525–57.

43. Cook TA, Davis RE. Cheek reconstruction. Op Tech Otolaryngol Head Neck Surg 1993;4:31–6.

44. Rapstine ED, Knaus WJ, Thornton JF. Simplifying cheek reconstruction: a review of over 400 cases. Plast Reconstr Surg 2012;129(6):1291–9.

45. Chu EA, Byrne PJ. Local flaps I: bilobed, rhombic, and cervicofacial. Facial Plast Surg Clin North Am 2009;17:349–60.

46. Menick FJ. Reconstruction of the cheek. Plast Reconstr Surg 2001;108:496–505.

47. Jowett N, Mlynarek AM. Reconstruction of cheek defects: a review of current techniques. Curr Opin Otolaryngol Head Neck Surg 2010;18:244–54.

48. Kroll SS, Reece GP, Robb G, et al. Deep-plane cervicofacial-rotation-advancement flap for recon-struction of large cheek defects. Plast Reconstr Surg 1994;94:88–93.

49. Tan ST, MacKinnon CA. Deep plane cervicofacial flap: a useful and versatile technique in head and neck surgery. Head Neck 2006;28:46–55.

50. Austen WG Jr, Parrett BM, Taghinia A, et al. The subcutaneous cervicofacial flap revisited. Ann Plast Surg 2009;62:149–53.

51. McLean JN, Carlson CW, Losken A. The pectoralis major myocutaneous flap revisited: a reliable technique for head and neck reconstruction. Ann Plast Surg 2010;64:570–3.

52. Ahmad QG, Navadgi S, Agarwal R, et al. Bipaddle pectoralis major myocutaneous flap in reconstructing full thickness defects of cheek: a review of 47 cases. J Plast Reconstr Aesthet Surg 2006;59:166–73.

53. Ozkan O, Mardini S, Chen HC, et al. Repair of buccal defects with anterolateral thigh flaps. Micro-surgery 2006;26:182–9.

54. Angelos PC, Downs BW. Options for the manage-ment of forehead and scalp defects. Facial Plast Surg Clin North Am 2009;17:379–93.

55. McCombe D, Donato R, Hofer S, et al. Free flaps in the treatment of locally advanced malignancy of the scalp and forehead. Ann Plast Surg 2002;48:600–6.

56. Beasley NJ, Gilbert RW, Gullane PJ, et al. Scalp and forehead reconstruction using free vascularized tissue transfer. Arch Facial Plast Surg 2004;6:16–20.

57. van Driel AA, Mureau MA, Goldstein DP, et al. Aesthetic and oncologic outcome after microsur-gical reconstruction of complex scalp and forehead defects after malignant tumor resection: an algo-rithm for treatment. Plast Reconstr Surg 2010;126:460–70.

58. Zinkernagel MS, Catalano E, Ammann-Rauch D. Free tarsal graft combined with skin transposition flap for full-thickness lower eyelid reconstruction. Ophthal Plast Reconstr Surg 2007;23:228–31.

59. Whitehouse GM, Francis IC. Eyelid reconstruction using a monopedicle flap and buccal mucosa: report of 15 cases. Aust N Z J Ophthalmol 1988;16:295–301.

60. Codner MA, McCord CD, Mjia JD, et al. Upper and lower eyelid. Plast Reconstr Surg 2010;126:231e–45e.

61. Tanaka A, Hatoko M, Tada H, et al. Histological evalu-ation of grafted hard palate mucosa in the reconstruc-tion of upper eyelid. Scand J Plast Reconstr Surg Hand Surg 2005;39:376–8.

62. Ito R, Fujiwara M, Nagasako R. Hard palate mucoper-iosteal graft for posterior lamellar reconstruction of the upper eyelid: histologic rationale. J Craniofac Surg 2007;18:684–90.

63. Wilscek G, Leatherbarrow B, Halliwell M, et al. The "RITE" use of the Fricke flap in periorbital recon-struction. Eye 2005;19:854–60.

64. Morley AM, deSousa JL, Selva D, et al. Techniques of upper eyelid reconstruction. Surv Ophthalmol 2010;55:256–71.

Nonmelanoma Skin Cancer of the Head and Neck: Prevention

Fatih Oghan, MD[a],*, Görkem Eskiizmir, MD[b],
Halis Unlu, MD[c], Cemal Cingi, MD[d]

KEYWORDS

- Nonmelanoma skin cancer • Head-neck • Tanning • Photoprotection • Summer season • UV

KEY POINTS

- Ultraviolet B (UVB) radiation is the main cause of photocarcinogenesis, sunburn, and immunosuppression.
- The amount of UVB is affected by geography (equatorial latitude, high altitude), season (spring, summer), meteorology (a sunny day without clouds), environment (ground reflections such as beach sand and sea), and time of day (midday between 10:00 AM and 4:00 PM).

INTRODUCTION

Nonmelanoma skin cancers (NMSCs) are the most commonly diagnosed cancers especially in the white race. The major etiologic factor for the development of NMSCs is the exposure to ultraviolet (UV) radiation (especially UVB and UVA radiation), which may cause DNA damage and genetic mutations in skin (Fig. 1).[1] Because of the detrimental effect of UV radiation, sun exposure is a high risk factor, especially for individuals who have phenotypic factors such as white or cream-white skin type, blue/green eyes, red or blond hair, or have freckles and moles. In addition, human papilloma virus, ionizing radiation, arsenic exposure, and genetic predisposition (such as xeroderma pigmentosum, albinism, or Muir-Torre syndrome) are the other important risk factors.[2]

A recent epidemiologic review about NMSCs has demonstrated that the incidence of NMSCs is increasing, and NMSCs are becoming a health care problem worldwide.[3] The investigators also highlighted that prevention and early detection are of paramount importance. The American Cancer Society emphasized that approximately 80% of all skin cancers are preventable.[4] The prevention of skin cancers can be managed by primary, secondary, and tertiary prevention strategies.

Primary prevention strategies include all the personal, institutional, and governmental efforts that provide the protection of the healthy population from the development of skin cancers.

Secondary prevention strategies include the early detection of skin cancers by performing total-body skin examination and involves case finding (incidental detection of a skin cancer in individuals who were seen for another medical problem or during routine check-up), screening (regular examination of high-risk individuals or population), and surveillance (periodic examination of patients who have suspicious lesions).[5]

In tertiary prevention, a regular and routine total-body skin examination is performed on patients who formerly had a diagnosis of skin cancer; thereby, a secondary skin cancer can be

Acknowledgment of Financial Support/Funding: None.
[a] Department of Otolaryngology, Head & Neck Surgery, Dumlupinar University, DPU Merkez Kampus, Tavsanli Yolu 10 km, Tıp Fakultesi, KBB AD, Kutahya 43270, Turkey; [b] Department of Otolaryngology, Head & Neck Surgery, Faculty of Medicine, Celal Bayar University, Manisa 45030, Turkey; [c] EKOL Hospital, Department of Otolaryngology, Head & Neck Surgery Hospital, 8019/16 street, Izmir, Turkey; [d] Department of Otorhinolaryngology, Head & Neck Surgery, Eskisehir Osmangazi University, Hasan Polatkan Street, Meselik 26020, Eskisehir, Turkey
* Corresponding author.
E-mail address: fatihoghan@hotmail.com

Facial Plast Surg Clin N Am 20 (2012) 515–523
http://dx.doi.org/10.1016/j.fsc.2012.08.005
1064-7406/12/$ – see front matter © 2012 Elsevier Inc. All rights reserved.

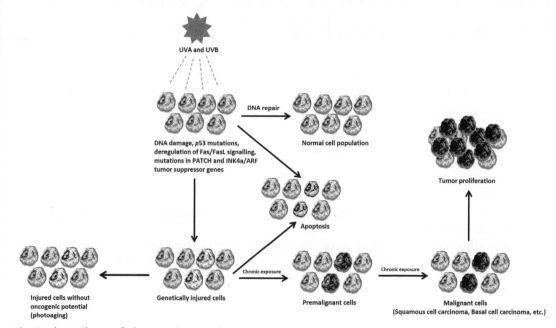

Fig. 1. The pathway of photocarcinogenesis.

detected and treated instantaneously, when it develops.

In this article, the importance and effectiveness of prevention efforts and strategies for skin cancers are reviewed.

PRIMARY PREVENTION STRATEGIES

Primary prevention strategies aim to avoid the development of NMSCs in the population and mainly include knowledge, behaviors, and attitudes about sun protection, chemoprevention, and public education programs.

Sun-Protection Behaviors and Clothing

The evidence has indicated that "intermittent" exposure to the sun increases the risk of development of basal cell carcinoma (BCC); however, squamous cell carcinoma (SCC) is strongly associated with continuing, chronic sun exposure. As solar UV radiation is the major etiologic factor for NMSCs, avoiding exposure to sunlight may lead to a remarkable reduction in prevalence. Sunlight includes different wavelengths, such as infrared and UV. The latter is part of the nonionizing electromagnetic spectrum and is divided into 3 spatial regions according to their wavelengths[6]:

1. Long-wave: UVA; 320–400 nm
2. Mid-wave: UVB; 290–320 nm
3. Short-wave: UVC; 200–290 nm

UV C is mutagenic for human skin; however, it does not reach the surface of the earth.

UV A comprises 90% to 95% of solar UV radiation and has a role in photoaging and immunosuppression; its role in photocarcinogenesis is controversial.[7–9]

UV B radiation is the main cause of photocarcinogenesis, sunburn, and immunosuppression.[9] The amount of UVB is affected by the following:

- Geography: equatorial latitude, high altitude
- Season: spring, summer
- Meteorology: a sunny day without clouds
- Environment: ground reflections, such as beach sand and sea
- Time of day: midday between 10:00 AM and 4:00 PM

The intensity of UV radiation (also called UV index) is forecasted daily to the public to warn of the hazardous effect of sun (Fig. 2). The UV index is an international standard measurement of the predicted UV radiation of a region and is presented on a scale between 1 and 11+ (Fig. 3). A high number indicates a greater risk of sunburn, especially for high-risk individuals.

Sun-protection behaviors and attitudes play an important role in the prevention of skin cancer. The recommendations about prevention from sun exposure are briefly presented in Box 1. Staying indoors to avoid midday sun, especially when the UV index is over 8, is very important for infants, children, adolescents, and even adults. In addition, seeking shade can be somewhat useful for sun protection; however, it does not provide

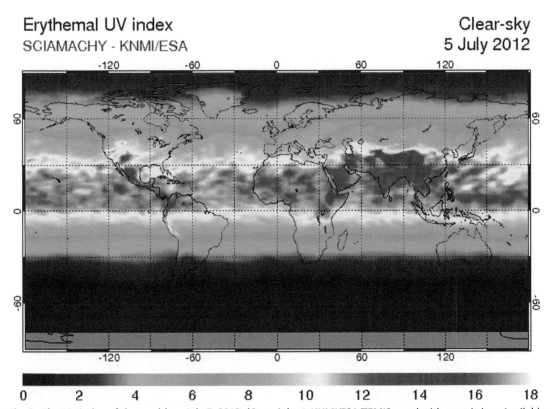

Fig. 2. The UV index of the world on July 5, 2012. (Copyright © KNMI/ESA/TEMIS; used with permission. Available at: www.temis.nl).

adequate protection from reflected and scattered UV radiation. Clothing is a simple, practical, and effective method for sun protection; however, several studies have demonstrated that most summer garments cannot provide adequate protection against the hazards of sunlight. Therefore, the authors recommend the use of UV-protective clothing items.[10] The UV-protection factor of a garment is a measure that demonstrates its ability to block solar UV radiation, and classified as:

Good: 15 to 24
Very good: 25 to 39
Excellent: 40 to 50 or greater

Various reasons may significantly influence the UV-protection factor of apparel textiles: fabric material and porosity, thickness, color, transparency, stretch, and presence of UV-protective absorbers. Therefore, UV-protective textile standards and guidelines have already been established for garment manufacturers and sun-aware consumers.[11,12]

Topical Sunscreen

Sunscreen was initially marketed in the 1920s in the United States and in the 1930s in Europe,

and has become a commercial product since then. To date, many sunscreen products have been manufactured with various combinations of sun-protective chemicals. Sunscreens can provide excellent protection against sunlight when applied appropriately and used responsibly; however, they are accepted as an adjunct technique to other types of sun-protection strategies.[13] They are mainly designed to prevent acute sunburn and tanning. In addition, it has been demonstrated that sunscreens can reduce the formation of actinic damage, solar keratoses, and NMSCs.[14–17]

An ideal topical sunscreen product should contain active sunscreen ingredients that are nontoxic and stable in the presence of light, water, and/or moisture, and provide good protection against sunlight, UVB and UVA radiation, scavenge-free radicals, and activate DNA repair systems to repair actinic damage.[18–20] The efficacy of a sunscreen product is denoted by sun protection factor (SPF), which reflects the protection against erythema that is mainly induced by UVB exposure. Sun protection factor basically indicates the ratio of the UVB radiation dose that produces minimal erythema on sunscreen-protected (skin cream thickness of 2 mg/cm^2)

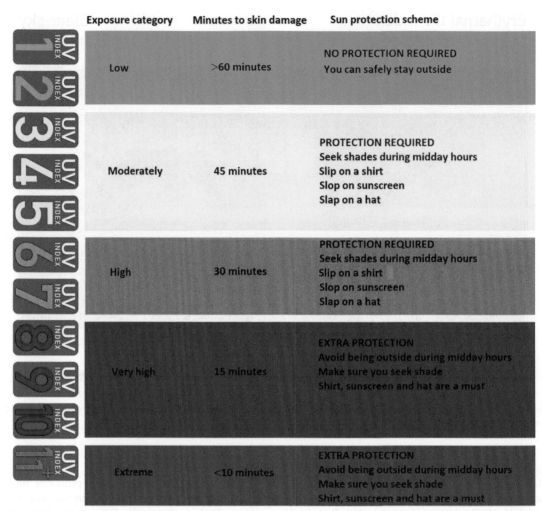

Exposure category	Minutes to skin damage	Sun protection scheme
Low	>60 minutes	**NO PROTECTION REQUIRED** You can safely stay outside
Moderately	45 minutes	**PROTECTION REQUIRED** Seek shades during midday hours Slip on a shirt Slop on sunscreen Slap on a hat
High	30 minutes	**PROTECTION REQUIRED** Seek shades during midday hours Slip on a shirt Slop on sunscreen Slap on a hat
Very high	15 minutes	**EXTRA PROTECTION** Avoid being outside during midday hours Make sure you seek shade Shirt, sunscreen and hat are a must
Extreme	<10 minutes	**EXTRA PROTECTION** Avoid being outside during midday hours Make sure you seek shade Shirt, sunscreen and hat are a must

Fig. 3. The scale of UV index. (*Adapted from* World Health Organization. Global Solar UV Index: A practical index of World Health Organization Library Catalogue. Geneva: World Health Organization, 2002.)

skin to the UVB radiation dose that produces minimal erythema on unprotected skin. Therefore, the efficiency of photoprotection is greater when the SPF value of a sunscreen product is higher. However, the relationship between SPF value and UVB radiation protection is not linear, which means that a twofold increase in SPF will not cause a twofold increase in UVB radiation protection. For example: a sunscreen with an SPF value of 15 can provide 94% protection against UVB radiation, whereas a sunscreen with an SPF value of 30 can provide 97% protection against UVB radiation. The main drawback of SPF is the photoprotective efficacy of a sunscreen against UVA, which may cause photoaging, immunosuppression, or DNA damage, is not indicated in this grading system. The water resistance of a sunscreen product is labeled with "water resistant (40 minutes)," which indicates protection of up to

40 minutes in continuous water exposure, and "water resistant (80 minutes)," which indicates a protection of up to 80 minutes in continuous water exposure. In addition, most of the recently manufactured sunscreen products contain multiple chemicals and different ingredients to provide broad-spectrum (against UVB and UVA) photoprotection. Ultimately, the American Academy of Dermatology recommends particularly the application of a sunscreen that is broad spectrum, water resistant, and has an SPF value of at least 30 to all exposed regions, such as head, neck, and extremities.[21]

The active ingredients of topical sunscreens are mainly classified as inorganic and organic chemical agents. Inorganic chemical agents act as a physical blocker by reflecting, scattering, and/or absorbing UV and infrared radiation. The major inorganic molecules that are used in sunscreens

---

Box 1
Sun-protection behaviors and attitudes

- Avoiding or minimizing exposure to the sun, especially between 10:00 AM and 4:00 PM

- Watching the daily UV index reports, and staying indoors when the sun exposure category is very high or extreme.

- Staying in the shade or using an umbrella.

- Wearing sunglasses that block 99% of UVA and UVB radiation.

- Avoiding indoor and outdoor tanning.

- Wearing sun-protective clothing (preferably UV protection factor 50+):

  ○ A bucket hat with at least a 3-inch brim or legionnaire cap.

  ○ Long-sleeved shirts and long clothing to the ankles, preferably

    ■ Dark-colored (such as black, navy blue) fabrics

    ■ Made of synthetic (especially polyester), denim, and wool materials

    ■ Tightly woven fibers

    ■ Dry materials

- Applying sunscreens with higher SPF (preferably 2 mg/cm^2 or 30 g for the whole body) at least 30 minutes before sun exposure; and reapplying after 90 to 120 minutes or after swimming, showering, toweling, or excessive sweating.

---

are zinc oxide and titanium dioxide. Although both titanium dioxide and zinc oxide have a photoprotective effect against UVB and UVA radiation; titanium dioxide is a better photoblocker for UVB, whereas zinc oxide provides better UVA protection. High-quality inorganic sunscreens are now manufactured by micronization and encapsulation; thereby, they are more cosmetically appealing and their protective efficacy against UV radiation increases remarkably.[22,23] Organic chemical agents principally show their photoprotective effect by absorbing UV radiation, and thereby, prevent penetration to the skin. They mainly contain 3 groups according to their protective characteristics against UVB and UVA radiation[20,24–26]:

1. UVB-absorbing sunscreens: cinnamates, p-aminobenzoate (PABA) derivatives, and salicylates, ensulizole, octocrylene.
2. UVA-absorbing sunscreens: avobenzone, ecamsule (terephthalylidene dicamphor sulfonic acid), meradimate (menthyl anthranilate).
3. Dual UVB/UVA absorbing sunscreens: camphor derivatives, oxybenzone.

Most of the topical sunscreens with an SPF value over 30 contain an inorganic and at least 2 organic chemical agents. In addition, other chemicals, such as vitamin C and E, which act as antioxidants and neutralize radical oxygen species generated by UV radiation, and aloe, which decreases the hazardous effects of UV radiation, are also used in several sunscreens.

The protective effect of topical sunscreens against sunburn has been demonstrated in humans.[26,27] In addition, Green and colleagues[28] reported favorable results in the prevention of actinic keratoses and SCC of the skin when topical sunscreens were used regularly and properly during sun exposure. In this study, people who applied broad-spectrum sunscreen with SPF value of 15+ to their sun-exposed skin (head, neck, arms, and hands) at least 3 to 4 days a week were compared with those who did not apply or applied fewer than 2 days a week. They observed a 40% reduction in SCC after 4.5 years; however, no significant benefit for BCC was demonstrated. Similarly, Van der Pols and colleagues[29] determined a decrease in the incidence of SCC without any significant difference in the incidence of BCC after regular application of sunscreens. Moreover, Vainio and colleagues[26] reviewed all the deliberations about the sunscreen and skin cancer that were held at the meeting of the International Agency for Research on Cancer at Lyon, France, from April 10 to 18, 2000. They declared that there was inadequate evidence that supports the preventive effect of sunscreens on the formation of BCC; on the other hand, sunscreens can reduce the development of actinic keratoses, which are a precursor of SCC. To highlight the cancer-preventive efficacy of sunscreens, large population-based, multicenter, randomized, double-blind, placebo-controlled, prospective trials are required.

The behavioral and attitudinal changes, including sunscreen application, are generally easy to perform and life saving; nevertheless, they are not widely accepted and practiced even in developed countries. In 1997, Hall and colleagues[30] aimed to examine the sun-protection behaviors in the US population and collected data from 10,048 white citizens. They determined that only 30% seek shade, 28% wear sun-protective clothes, and 32% apply sunscreen; therefore, they concluded that sun-protective behaviors are practiced in a limited percentage of the US population. In 2011, Buller and colleagues[31] reviewed the collected national and statewide behavioral surveys about the sun-protection behaviors in the US population. They determined that a minority of adults (30%) routinely engaged in sun-protection behaviors. In addition, a high rate of sunburning (69%) and low rate of sun-protection behaviors (40%) were detected in adolescents. Unfortunately, both of these studies demonstrate that sun-protection behaviors have not changed significantly in the past 2 decades in the US population. In addition, Stanton and colleagues[32] investigated the efficacy and practice of primary prevention of skin cancer in Australia. This study revealed that the most commonly practiced sun-protection behavior in children, adolescents, and adults was sunscreen application. On the other hand, sun-protection clothing and attitudes were inadequate. They emphasized that public education interventions did not change people's sun behaviors and attitudes, and the relationships between sun protection and reduction in skin cancers, and tanning/sunbathing and increase in skin cancer were poorly understood, even with the awareness of the population about the potential risks of solar UV radiation was accomplished.

Chemoprevention

Sun-protection behaviors and regular application of sunscreen are recommended as a primary prevention method; however, additional preventive interventions, such as chemoprevention, are generally required, especially for high-risk patients. Chemoprevention is a promising strategy that may provide inhibition and/or reversal of the development of skin cancer. An ideal chemopreventive agent should be safe with or without minimal toxicity and have a significant efficacy in decreasing the incidence of skin cancer. Topical and oral forms of natural, synthetic, or biologic chemical agents are used for chemoprevention. The most popular chemical agents that have proven of potential efficacy for chemoprevention are[33–37] the following:

1. Retinol and retinoids
2. Difluoromethylornithine
3. Green tea polyphenols
4. Cyclo-oxygenase-2 inhibitors
5. T4 endonuclease V (Dimericine)
6. Photolyase
7. Lycopene
8. Silymarin
9. Genestein
10. Vitamin D

All of the chemopreventive agents mentioned may influence and inhibit the process of photocarcinogenesis in different stages[38]; however, retinoids and retinol are the only chemical agents that have the proven to have a chemopreventive effect of NMSCs in humans. The mechanisms that may play a role in chemopreventive properties of retinoids are inhibition of cell growth, induction of apoptosis and differentiation, modification of extracellular adhesion molecules, and protooncogenes.[39–41] The Southwest Skin Cancer Prevention Study Group examined the chemopreventive effect of retinol (a daily supplementation of 25,000 IU) in moderate-risk patients in a randomized, double-blind, controlled study. They demonstrated that retinol supplementation reduces the development of SCC; however, it is not beneficial for the prevention of BCC.[42] In a different study, they also investigated the chemopreventive effect of retinol and isotretinoin in high-risk patients. Unfortunately, no beneficial chemopreventive effect was found with retinol and isotretinin.[43] Similarly, a long-term (approximately 12 years), randomized, double-blind, placebo-controlled clinical trial indicated that beta carotene supplementation (50 mg/d) is not beneficial for the prevention of the development of an NMSC (both BCC and SCC) among healthy well-nourished men.[44] In addition, Greenberg and colleagues[45] did not find a significant reduction in the development of BCC and/or SCC in patients who had a history of previous NMSC after treatment with beta carotene (50 mg/d). On the other hand, Kraemer and colleagues[46] investigated the chemopreventive effects of retinoids in 5 patients with xeroderma pigmentosum to whom oral isotretinoin at a dosage of 2 mg/kg/d was applied for 2 years. They observed a statistically significant difference when the mean number of NMSCs before (mean: 24) and after (mean: 5) treatment were compared. Moreover, the tumor frequency increased a mean of 8.5-fold after the discontinuation of the drug. Therefore, they concluded that high-dose oral isotretinoin is a beneficial drug for the chemoprophylaxis of skin cancers in patients with xeroderma pigmentosum; however, they also emphasized that this treatment may cause some side effects, such as mucocutaneous toxicities, and liver-function and skeletal abnormalities. Therefore, chemoprevention with systemic retinoid treatment is generally recommended when the benefits overshadow the potential risks and complications, and almost always applied in conjunction with another prevention intervention for NMSC. Ultimately, Prado and colleagues[37] reviewed the indications of retinoids for NMSC chemoprophylaxis and signified the candidates for this treatment who are

- Patients who had chronic immunosuppression owing to organ transplantation, lymphoma, or leukemia, or are carriers of human immunodeficiency virus
- Patients with psoriasis
- Patients who have a history of previous NMSC or photochemotherapy (PUVA) treatment
- Patients with radiation-induced NMSC
- Patients with xeroderma pigmentosum, nevoid BCC syndrome, Bazex syndrome, Rombo syndrome, or epidermodysplasia syndrome

Other agents, difluoromethylornithine, T4 endonuclease V, curcumin, and isoflavone genestein, appear safe; however, clinical trials that would establish their efficacy in human beings have not been completed yet.

Lycopene, green tea (epigallocatechin gallate), grape seed extract, and silymarin have been shown to be effective in experimental studies.[33]

Chemical agents that have been disproved for NMSC chemoprevention are the following[47,48]:

- Vitamin E (oral alfa-tocopherol 400 IU/d)
- Selenium (oral selenium 200 μg/d)

SECONDARY PREVENTION

Secondary prevention principally aims for early detection of a skin cancer by total-body skin examinations in individuals without a history of skin cancer or otherwise at high risk. Ferrini and colleagues[49] emphasized that a total-body skin examination is a noninvasive and reliable (with a sensitivity of 89% to 97%) screening procedure when performed by a physician who is experienced in examinations of skin lesions and cancers. Theoretically, a regular and routine total-body skin examination may increase the detection of early skin cancers; thereby early medical or surgical treatments can be performed with relatively low morbidity and mortality. Nevertheless, the US Preventive Services Task Force stated that although skin cancer screening is a promising strategy for the reduction of skin cancers, the evidence is inadequate to demonstrate the efficacy of skin cancer screening for the early detection of skin cancers.[50,51] However, a recently reported epidemiologic, prospective clinical trial, also named the SCREEN Project (Skin Cancer Research to Provide Evidence for Effectiveness of Screening in Northern Germany), from Germany demonstrated that a large-scale systematic skin cancer screening program is feasible.[52] In this study, 43,583 NMSCs (31,258 BCCs and 11,682 SCCs) and 7147 malignant melanomas were detected between 1999 and 2006. In addition, they observed a significant reduction in melanoma mortality (men: observed 0.79/100,000 and expected 2.00/100,000; women: observed 0.66/100,000 and expected 1.30/100,000) 5 years after the SCREEN project. Although the results of this study are very promising, there are some limitations, such as the participation rate is low (19%) and the level of evidence is not high, because it is not a randomized controlled study.

TERTIARY PREVENTION

Tertiary prevention mainly delays with the early detection of a new NMSC in patients with a history of a previous skin cancer by periodic total-body skin examinations. The risk of development of a subsequent NMSC in patients with a history of previous NMSC is relatively high. Marcil and Stern[53] reviewed the literature and reported that 18% of patients with a history of a previous SCC developed a new SCC and 44% of patients with a history of a previous BCC developed a new BCC at 3 years. Therefore, a regular, routine follow-up of patients with NMSC for at least 4 years with reexaminations at least every 3 months during the first year and every 6 months thereafter is recommended.[54]

SUMMARY

Skin cancers are becoming a health care problem worldwide. The development of skin cancer can be prevented by photoprotection, which should begin in infancy and childhood. Therefore, health care providers should inform the parents and adults about the hazardous effects of sun exposure and protection interventions. Sun-protection behaviors, including topical sunscreen application, are generally cost-effective and can reduce the development of NMSC; however, they are not practiced widely. Therefore, the population should be educated about the sun-protection behaviors with governmental campaigns and topical sunscreen application should be encouraged. Chemoprevention is a promising adjunct strategy especially for high-risk patients. Chemopreventive agents may inhibit the development of skin cancer by targeting different steps of photocarcinogenesis; however, clinical trials with high levels of evidence are required. Skin cancer screening is a promising strategy that may have a wide acceptance in the future.

REFERENCES

1. Melnikova VO, Ananthaswamy HN. Cellular and molecular events leading to the development of skin cancer. Mutat Res 2005;571:91–106.

2. Madan V, Lear JT, Szeimies RM. Nonmelanoma skin cancer. Lancet 2010;375:673–85.

3. Lomas A, Leonardi-Bee J, Bath-Hextall F. A systematic review of worldwide incidence of nonmelanoma skin cancer. Br J Dermatol 2012;166:1069–80.

4. American Cancer Society. Facts and figures. Atlanta (GA): American Cancer Society; 2007.

5. Mahon SM. Skin cancer prevention: education and public health issues. Semin Oncol Nurs 2003;19:52–61.

6. Jou PC, Feldman RJ, Tomecki KJ. UV protection and sunscreens: what to tell patients. Cleve Clin J Med 2012;79:427–36.

7. Coldiron BM. The UV Index: a weather report for skin. Clin Dermatol 1998;16:441–6.

8. Nghiem DX, Kazimi N, Clydesdale G, et al. Ultraviolet a radiation suppresses an established immune response: implications for sunscreen design. J Invest Dermatol 2001;117:1193–9.

9. Katiyar SK. UV-induced immune suppression and photocarcinogenesis: chemoprevention by dietary botanical agents. Cancer Lett 2007;255:1–11.

10. Hoffmann K, Laperre J, Avermaete A, et al. Defined UV protection by apparel textiles. Arch Dermatol 2001;137:1089–94.

11. Gambichler T, Laperre J, Hoffmann K. The European standard for sun-protective clothing: EN 13758. J Eur Acad Dermatol Venereol 2006;20:125–30.

12. Hatch KL. American standards for UV-protective textiles. Recent Results Cancer Res 2002;160:42–7.

13. Green AC, Williams GM. Point: sunscreen use is a safe and effective approach to skin cancer prevention. Cancer Epidemiol Biomarkers Prev 2007;16:1921–2.

14. Thompson SC, Jolley D, Marks R. Reduction of solar keratoses by regular sunscreen use. N Engl J Med 1993;329:1147–51.

15. Naylor MF, Boyd A, Smith DW, et al. High sun protection factor sunscreens in the suppression of actinic neoplasia. Arch Dermatol 1995;131:170–5.

16. Naylor MF, Farmer KC. The case for sunscreens. A review of their use in preventing actinic damage and neoplasia. Arch Dermatol 1997;133:1146–54.

17. Gordon LG, Scuffham PA, van der Pols JC, et al. Regular sunscreen use is a cost-effective approach to skin cancer prevention in subtropical settings. J Invest Dermatol 2009;129:2766–71.

18. Rapaport MJ, Rapaport V. Preventive and therapeutic approaches to short- and long-term sun damaged skin. Clin Dermatol 1998;16:429–39.

19. Scherschun L, Lim HW. Photoprotection by sunscreens. Am J Clin Dermatol 2001;2:131–4.

20. Sambandan DR, Ratner D. Sunscreens: an overview and update. J Am Acad Dermatol 2011;64:748–58.

21. American Academy of Dermatology. Melanoma. Available at: www.aad.org/media-resources/stats-and-facts/conditions/melanoma/melanoma. Accessed December 8, 2011.

22. Villalobos-Hernandez JR, Muller-Goymann CC. Novel nanoparticulate carrier system based on carnauba wax and decyl oleate for the dispersion of inorganic sunscreens in aqueous media. Eur J Pharm Biopharm 2005;60:113–22.

23. Villalobos-Hernandez JR, Muller-Goymann CC. Sun protection enhancement of titanium dioxide crystals by the use of carnauba wax nanoparticles: the synergistic interaction between organic and inorganic sunscreens at nanoscale. Int J Pharm 2006;322:161–70.

24. Lautenschlager S, Wulf HC, Pittelkow MR. Photoprotection. Lancet 2007;370:528–37.

25. González S, Fernández-Lorente M, Gilaberte-Calzada Y. The latest on skin photoprotection. Clin Dermatol 2008;26:614–26.

26. Vainio H, Miller AB, Bianchini F. An international evaluation of the cancer-preventive potential of sunscreens. Int J Cancer 2000;88:838–42.

27. Berwick M. Counterpoint: sunscreen use is a safe and effective approach to skin cancer prevention. Cancer Epidemiol Biomarkers Prev 2007;16:1923–4.

28. Green A, Williams G, Neale R, et al. Daily sunscreen application and betacarotene supplementation in prevention of basal-cell and squamous-cell carcinomas of the skin: a randomised controlled trial. Lancet 1999;354:723–9.

29. van der Pols JC, Williams GM, Pandeya N, et al. Prolonged prevention of squamous cell carcinoma of the skin by regular sunscreen use. Cancer Epidemiol Biomarkers Prev 2006;15:2546–8.

30. Hall HI, May DS, Lew RA, et al. Sun protection behaviors of the U.S. white population. Prev Med 1997;26:401–7.

31. Buller DB, Cokkinides V, Hall HI, et al. Prevalence of sunburn, sun protection, and indoor tanning behaviors among Americans: review from national surveys and case studies of 3 states. J Am Acad Dermatol 2011;65:S114–23.

32. Stanton WR, Janda M, Baade PD, et al. Primary prevention of skin cancer: a review of sun protection in Australia and internationally. Health Promot Int 2004;19:369–78.

33. Stratton SP, Dorr RT, Alberts DS. The state-of-the-art in chemoprevention of skin cancer. Eur J Cancer 2000;36:1292–7.

34. Einspahr JG, Stratton SP, Bowden GT, et al. Chemoprevention of human skin cancer. Crit Rev Oncol Hematol 2002;41:269–85.

35. Wright TI, Spencer JM, Flowers FP. Chemoprevention of nonmelanoma skin cancer. J Am Acad Dermatol 2006;54:933–46.

36. Uliasz A, Spencer JM. Chemoprevention of skin cancer and photoaging. Clin Dermatol 2004;22:178–82.

37. Prado R, Francis SO, Mason MN, et al. Nonmelanoma skin cancer chemoprevention. Dermatol Surg 2011;37:1566–78.

38. Camp WL, Turnham JW, Athar M, et al. New agents for prevention of ultraviolet-induced nonmelanoma skin cancer. Semin Cutan Med Surg 2011;30:6–13.

39. Breitman TR, Selonick SE, Collins SJ. Induction of differentiation of the human promyelocytic leukemia cell line (HL-60) by retinoic acid. Proc Natl Acad Sci U S A 1980;77:2936–40.

40. Schule R, Rangarajan P, Yang N, et al. Retinoic acid is a negative regulator of AP-1-responsive genes. Proc Natl Acad Sci U S A 1991;88:6092–6.

41. Mrass P, Rendl M, Mildner M, et al. Retinoic acid increases the expression of p53 and proapoptotic caspases and sensitizes keratinocytes to apoptosis: a possible explanation for tumor preventive action of retinoids. Cancer Res 2004;64:6542–8.

42. Moon TE, Levine N, Cartmel B, et al. Effect of retinol in preventing squamous cell skin cancer in moderate-risk subjects: a randomized, double-blind, controlled trial. Southwest Skin Cancer Prevention Study Group. Cancer Epidemiol Biomarkers Prev 1997;6:949–56.

43. Levine N, Moon TE, Cartmel B, et al. Trial of retinol and isotretinoin in skin cancer prevention: a randomized, double-blind, controlled trial. Southwest Skin Cancer Prevention Study Group. Cancer Epidemiol Biomarkers Prev 1997;6:957–61.

44. Frieling UM, Schaumberg DA, Kupper TS, et al. A randomized, 12-year primary-prevention trial of beta carotene supplementation for nonmelanoma skin cancer in the physician's health study. Arch Dermatol 2000;136:179–84.

45. Greenberg ER, Baron JA, Stukel TA, et al. A clinical trial of beta carotene to prevent basal-cell and squamous-cell cancers of the skin. The Skin Cancer Prevention Study Group. N Engl J Med 1990;323:789–95.

46. Kraemer KH, DiGiovanna JJ, Moshell AN, et al. Prevention of skin cancer in xeroderma pigmentosum with the use of oral isotretinoin. N Engl J Med 1988;318:1633–7.

47. Werninghaus K, Meydani M, Bhawan J, et al. Evaluation of the photoprotective effect of oral vitamin E supplementation. Arch Dermatol 1994;130:1257–61.

48. Duffield-Lillico AJ, Slate EH, Reid ME, et al. Selenium supplementation and secondary prevention of nonmelanoma skin cancer in a randomized trial. J Natl Cancer Inst 2003;95:1477–81.

49. Ferrini RL, Perlman M, Hill L. American College of Preventive Medicine policy statement: screening for skin cancer. Am J Prev Med 1998;14:80–2.

50. US Preventive Services Task Force. Screening for skin cancer: recommendations and rationale. Am J Prev Med 2001;20:44–6.

51. Wolff T, Tai E, Miller T. Screening for skin cancer: an update of the evidence for the U.S. Preventive Services Task Force. Ann Intern Med 2009;150:194–8.

52. Breitbart EW, Waldmann A, Nolte S, et al. Systematic skin cancer screening in Northern Germany. J Am Acad Dermatol 2012;66:201–11.

53. Marcil I, Stern RS. Risk of developing a subsequent nonmelanoma skin cancer in patients with a history of nonmelanoma skin cancer: a critical review of the literature and meta-analysis. Arch Dermatol 2000;136:1524–30.

54. Frankel DH, Hanusa BH, Zitelli JA. New primary nonmelanoma skin cancer in patients with a history of squamous cell carcinoma of the skin. Implications and recommendations for follow-up. J Am Acad Dermatol 1992;26:720–6.

Index

Note: Page numbers of article titles are in **boldface** type.

A

Abbe-Sabattini flap, in lip reconstruction, 500
Aborizing vessels, basal cell carcinoma and, 424–425
    as pigmented hallmark, 426–427
Actinic keratosis (AK), afamelanotide for, 451
  Bowenoid, 429
  cheilitis, 429
  clinical findings in, 428–429
  dermoscopic findings in, 429–430
  description of, 427
  development into squamous cell carcinoma,
    429, 432–433
  erythematous, 428
  histopathology of, 428–429
  keratotic, 428–429
  lichen planus–like, 428
  pigmented, 429–430
  reflectance confocal microscopy findings in, 430
  topical 5-FU for, 450
  UV-induced carcinogenesis in, 438
Advancement flap, in forehead reconstruction, 507
  in nose reconstruction, 495
Aesthetic units, facial, 493
Aesthetics, of facial appearance, reconstructive
  surgery for, **493–513.** See also *Reconstructive*
  surgery.
Afamelanotide (CUV1647), for nonmelanoma skin
  cancer, 447, 451
Alar-facial junction, basal cell carcinoma on, surgical
  excision of, 460–461
Anesthesia, for MMS, 463
  for surgical excision, of nonmelanoma skin
    cancer, 458–459
Anterolateral thigh flap, in cheek reconstruction,
  506
  in forehead reconstruction, 507
  in lip reconstruction, 500
Antioxidants, in topical sunscreen, 519
Apoptosis, in nonmelanoma skin cancer, 441
Arterial blood supply, in cheek reconstruction,
  505–506
  in lip reconstruction, 497, 502
As prognostic risk factor, burn scar, for
  nonmelanoma skin cancer, 458
  degree of differentiation, for nonmelanoma skin
    cancer, 457
  lesion size, for nonmelanoma skin cancer,
    456–457
A-T flap, in forehead reconstruction, 507–509

Attitudes, sun-protection, for nonmelanoma skin
  cancer prevention, 516–517, 519
Atypical fibroxanthoma (AFX), of head and neck,
  484, 486
Australia, nonmelanoma skin cancer in, economic
  burden of, 421
    incidence of, 415, 420

B

Basal cell carcinoma (BCC), aborizing vessels and,
  424–425
    as pigmented hallmark, 426–427
  as nonmelanoma skin cancer, 416, 419
  basosquamous, 424–425
  clinical findings in, 424–426, 428
  cyclopamine for, 451
  cystic, 425–426
  cytokines for, 451
  dermoscopic findings in, 426–428
  etiology of, 416
  fibroepithelioma of Pinkus as, 425
  hairpin vessels surrounding, 426–427
  histopathological subtypes of, 416, 425–426
  histopathology of, 426, 428
  imiquimod for, 450
  incidence of, 420
  incomplete excision of, controversial
    management of, 467–468
  infiltrative, 424–426
  keratocanthoma, 426–427
  laser therapy for, 450
  morpheaform, 424–426
  multiple face and neck, excision with MMS,
    463, 465
  narrow-margin elliptical excision of, 459–460
  nodular, 424, 426
  on alar-facial junction, surgical excision of,
    460–461
  on nasolabial fold, excision with MMS, 463, 465
  on nose, surgical excision of, 460–461
  on scalp, surgical excision of, 459–460
  photodynamic therapy for, 449
  pigmented, aborizing vessels as hallmark of,
    426–427
  pigmented nodular, 424, 426
  platelet-derived growth factor in, 441–442
  prevention of. See *Prevention strategies.*
  reflectance confocal microscopy findings in,
    427–428

Facial Plast Surg Clin N Am 20 (2012) 525–536
http://dx.doi.org/10.1016/S1064-7406(12)00128-9
1064-7406/12/$ – see front matter © 2012 Elsevier Inc. All rights reserved.

United States Postal Service

Statement of Ownership, Management, and Circulation
(All Periodicals Publications Except Requester Publications)

1. Publication Title	2. Publication Number	3. Filing Date
Facial Plastic Surgery Clinics of North America	0 1 3 - 1 2 2	9/14/12

4. Issue Frequency	5. Number of Issues Published Annually	6. Annual Subscription Price
Feb, May, Aug, Nov	4	$359.00

7. Complete Mailing Address of Known Office of Publication (Not printer) (Street, city, county, state, and ZIP+4®)

Elsevier Inc.
360 Park Avenue South
New York, NY 10010-1710

Contact Person
Stephen Bushing

Telephone (Include area code)
215-239-3688

8. Complete Mailing Address of Headquarters or General Business Office of Publisher (Not printer)

Elsevier Inc., 360 Park Avenue South, New York, NY 10010-1710

9. Full Names and Complete Mailing Addresses of Publisher, Editor, and Managing Editor (Do not leave blank)

Publisher (Name and complete mailing address)

Kim Murphy, Elsevier, Inc., 1600 John F. Kennedy Blvd. Suite 1800, Philadelphia, PA 19103-2899

Editor (Name and complete mailing address)

Joanne Husovski, Elsevier, Inc., 1600 John F. Kennedy Blvd. Suite 1800, Philadelphia, PA 19103-2899

Managing Editor (Name and complete mailing address)

Barbara Cohen - Kligerman, Elsevier, Inc., 1600 John F. Kennedy Blvd. Suite 1800, Philadelphia, PA 19103-2899

10. Owner (Do not leave blank. If the publication is owned by a corporation, give the name and address of the corporation immediately followed by the names and addresses of all stockholders owning or holding 1 percent or more of the total amount of stock. If not owned by a corporation, give the names and addresses of the individual owners. If owned by a partnership or other unincorporated firm, give its name and address as well as those of each individual owner. If the publication is published by a nonprofit organization, give its name and address.)

Full Name	Complete Mailing Address
Wholly owned subsidiary of	1600 John F. Kennedy Blvd, Ste. 1800
Reed/Elsevier, US holdings	Philadelphia, PA 19103-2899

11. Known Bondholders, Mortgagees, and Other Security Holders Owning or Holding 1 Percent or More of Total Amount of Bonds, Mortgages, or Other Securities. If none, check box ☐ None

Full Name	Complete Mailing Address
N/A	

12. Tax Status (For completion by nonprofit organizations authorized to mail at nonprofit rates) (Check one)
The purpose, function, and nonprofit status of this organization and the exempt status for federal income tax purposes:
☐ Has Not Changed During Preceding 12 Months
☐ Has Changed During Preceding 12 Months (Publisher must submit explanation of change with this statement)

PS Form 3526, September 2007 (Page 1 of 3 (Instructions Page 3)) PSN 7530-01-000-9931 PRIVACY NOTICE: See our Privacy policy in www.usps.com

---

13. Publication Title	14. Issue Date for Circulation Data Below
Facial Plastic Surgery Clinics of North America	August 2012

15. Extent and Nature of Circulation		Average No. Copies Each Issue During Preceding 12 Months	No. Copies of Single Issue Published Nearest to Filing Date
a. Total Number of Copies (Net press run)		661	597
b. Paid Circulation (By Mail and Outside the Mail)	(1) Mailed Outside-County Paid Subscriptions Stated on PS Form 3541. (Include paid distribution above nominal rate, advertiser's proof copies, and exchange copies)	344	324
	(2) Mailed In-County Paid Subscriptions Stated on PS Form 3541 (Include paid distribution above nominal rate, advertiser's proof copies, and exchange copies)		
	(3) Paid Distribution Outside the Mails Including Sales Through Dealers and Carriers, Street Vendors, Counter Sales, and Other Paid Distribution Outside USPS®	64	73
	(4) Paid Distribution by Other Classes Mailed Through the USPS (e.g. First-Class Mail®)		
c. Total Paid Distribution (Sum of 15b (1), (2), (3), and (4))	▲	408	397
d. Free or Nominal Rate Distribution (By Mail and Outside the Mail)	(1) Free or Nominal Rate Outside-County Copies Included on PS Form 3541	74	80
	(2) Free or Nominal Rate In-County Copies Included on PS Form 3541		
	(3) Free or Nominal Rate Copies Mailed at Other Classes Through the USPS (e.g. First-Class Mail)		
	(4) Free or Nominal Rate Distribution Outside the Mail (Carriers or other means)		
e. Total Free or Nominal Rate Distribution (Sum of 15d (1), (2), (3) and (4))	▲	74	80
f. Total Distribution (Sum of 15c and 15e)	▲	482	477
g. Copies not Distributed (See instructions to publishers #4 (page 83))	▲	179	120
h. Total (Sum of 15f and g)	▲	661	597
i. Percent Paid (15c divided by 15f times 100)		84.65%	83.23%

16. Publication of Statement of Ownership

If the publication is a general publication, publication of this statement is required. Will be printed in the November 2012 issue of this publication. ☐ Publication not required

17. Signature and Title of Editor, Publisher, Business Manager, or Owner

Stephen R. Bushing
Stephen R. Bushing Inventory/Distribution Coordinator

Date
September 14, 2012

I certify that all information furnished on this form is true and complete. I understand that anyone who furnishes false or misleading information on this form or who omits material or information requested on the form may be subject to criminal sanctions (including fines and imprisonment) and/or civil sanctions (including civil penalties).

PS Form 3526, September 2007 (Page 2 of 3)

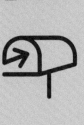

Moving?

Make sure your subscription
moves with you!

To notify us of your new address, find your **Clinics Account Number** (located on your mailing label above your name), and contact customer service at:

Email: journalscustomerservice-usa@elsevier.com

800-654-2452 (subscribers in the U.S. & Canada)
314-447-8871 (subscribers outside of the U.S. & Canada)

Fax number: 314-447-8029

Elsevier Health Sciences Division
Subscription Customer Service
3251 Riverport Lane
Maryland Heights, MO 63043

To ensure uninterrupted delivery of your subscription, please notify us at least 4 weeks in advance of move.

Printed and bound by CPI Group (UK) Ltd, Croydon, CR0 4YY

03/10/2024

01040346-0009